THA OMAD DIET COOKING BOOK 2022

A meal a day: a guide to losing weight, boosting energy, and your immune system with 180 delicious nutritional recipes.

D1567319

ONAROM

DISCLAIMER OF LIABILITY

This publication contains the views and ideas of its author. It aims to provide useful and informative material on the topics covered in the publication. It is sold with the understanding that the author and publisher are not engaged in providing medical, health care, or other personal professional services in the book. The reader should consult with their physician, health care practitioner, or other competent professional before adopting any suggestions in this book or drawing any conclusions. The author and publisher expressly disclaim any liability for any liability, loss, or risk, personal or otherwise, arising, directly or indirectly, from the use and application of any content in this book.

1 BONIATO ÑOCCHI
WITH BROCCOLI

2 CANEDERLI WITH CHICORY
AND SPINACH

3 THAI PADS

4 WHOLE PASTA WITH
LETTUCE PESTO

5 WHOLE BUTTERFLIES WITH
ONION AND GREEN OLIVES

6 UDON WITH PEANUT
SAUCE AND SESAME

7 SOFT PASTA AND CHICKPEAS

9 SPAGHETTI OF SPELLED WITH CREAM
OF LEEK AND CHICKPEAS WITH WHEAT
PAPER ARTICHOKE PASTA

11 TAGLIOLINI WITH FENNEL
WITH LEMON AND TEMPEH
CRUMBLE

12 FUSILLI DRIED ANACHARD TOMATOES

13 FETTUCCINE EDAMAME
WITH PUMPKIN, LENTILS, AND
WALNUTS

14 PENNE WITH VEGETABLE
SOY SAUCE WITH SAFFRON
CREAM

15 WHOLE SPAGHETTI WITH
CHICKPEAS AND PLUMS

16 WHOLE SPAGHETTI WITH
AUBERGINES WITH WALNUTS
AND BLACK OLIVES

17 WHOLE PASTA WITH
PUMPKIN ESCAPE

18 POTATO GNOCCHI WITH
PEAS AND BASIL PASTA

19 TAGLIATELLE WITH
CARROT AND BASIL SAUCE

20 TAGLIATELLE WITH
ARUGULA AND CASHEW PESTO

21 SPAGHETTI WITH SADDLE BACK WITH RIBS AND DRIED TOMATOES

22 WHOLE PASTA WITH CHESTNUT AND HAZELNUT BEACH SAUCE

23 FAST COLD AND CREAMY VEGETABLE PASTA

24 MALTAGLIATI WITH CHESTNUT AND PUMPKIN RAGU

25 WHOLE WHEAT HELL WITH EDAMAME

26 PLEUROTUS MUSHROOMS FOR FREE

27 ROASTED RED POTATOES WITH HERBS AND CORN

28 INSPECTED FENNELS TURMERIC WITH POTATOES AND ONIONS

29 FENNEL PIZZAIOLA

30 WINTER VEGETABLES BAKED
WITH 4-FLAVORED SAUCE

31 ISABELLA BAKED PASTA

32 SICILIAN CAKE

33 TUSCAN RAVIOLI

34 CANADIAN OAT FLOUR
COOKIES

35 IRISH OAT DONUT

36 SWEET OAT CREAM WITH
WILD BERRIES

37 SWEET OAT CREAM WITH ORANGE

38 SWEET OAT CREAM WITH
CHESTNUTS

39 SWEET OAT CREAM
WITH STRAWBERRY AND GRAPES

40 SWEET OAT CREAM
WITH APPLES AND PINIONS

**41 SCOTTISH STYLE
SWEET OAT CREAM**

42 BULGARIAN OAT CAKE

**43 MALTAGLIATI OAT FLOUR
WITH FRESH GRASS, BACON,
AND PEAS**

44 CAVATELLI WITH MUSHROOMS

**45 POTATO CREAM WITH
VEGETABLES**

**46 LEEK CREAM AND
CHESTNUTS**

**47 FETTUCCINE
ALL'ARRABBIATA WITH
ARTICHOKES**

48 FETTUCCINE WITH TRUFFLE

49 MEXICAN CAULIFLOWER RICE

**50 GOCKS OF CHINESE RICE WITH
VEGETABLES, SHIITAKE, AND
ALMONDS**

51 HIGH BANANA IN
ZALAMERO PROTEIN

52 INTEGRAL BRETZEL

53 BREAKFAST WITH PUMPKIN BREAD

54 MEDITERRANEAN OMELET

55 CREAMY OAT FLOUR WITH
BANANA

56 PAN OF SHRIMPS

57 TOMORROW "GRILL"

58 BREAKFAST WITH MEAT

59 ROLLED OATS, APPLES, AND SPICES

60 OAT FLOUR, APPLE, AND
BAKED CINNAMON

61 YOGURT BANANA ALMOND

62 BAKED EGGS BASIL AND TOMATO

63 BLUEBERRY AND MAPLE
OATMEAL

64 BUCATINI AMATRICIANA

65 LENTIL CREAM

66 POTATO CREAM WITH
VEGETABLES

67 LEEK AND CHESTNUT CREAM

68 ANGRY FETTUCCINE
WITH ARTICHOKES

69 FETTUCCINE
ARTICHOKES AND BACON

70 GREEN FETTUCCINE
WITH CHICKEN AND
CHILEAN SAUCE

71 RADICCHIO RAVIOLI
AND RICOTTA

72 ZUCCHINI STUFFED WITH BEEF

73 RIGATONI WITH MEATBALLS

74 BEAN SOUP HAT

75 PASTA AND BEANS

76 CABBAGE ROLLS

77 MUFFINS FOR EGG BREAKFAST

78 EASY AND DELICIOUS
SAUSAGE FRITTATA

79 ROASTED VEGETABLES
WITH PEANUT SAUCE

80 CAULIFLOWER CREAM
SAUCE WITH SAUCE

81 WHITE PIZZA WITH BROCCOLI CRUST

82 BEANS WITH GARLIC

83 GARLIC ZOODLES

84 MEDITERRANEAN SALMON

85 PASTA WITH CHICKEN
PESTO WITHOUT FAT AND
VEGETABLES

86 LIGHT SMOKE WITH VEGETABLES

87 PUMPKIN AND PUMPKIN SOUP

102 CHILDREN WITH ALGAE

103 GÂTEAU OF POTATOES

104 MINI QUICHE OF PUMPKIN
WITH MINT AND PISTACHIOS

105 YELLOW POTATO CAKE

106 POTATO CRUMBLE

107 FLAN OF TUNA AND POTATOES

108 FRYING TOAST OF FRENCH FRIES

109 CROQUETTES OF
POTATOES WITH
CURRENT HEART

110 HALF SLEEVE OF
TUNA AND OLIVES

111 CHICKEN WITH PEPPERS

112 STUFFED BREAST
WITH CHICKEN
BREAST

113 STRIPS OF CHICKEN
SAFFRON AND PUMPKIN

114 BAKED FRITTATA WITH POTATOES AND ONIONS

115 CASHEW CHEESE WITH BLUEBERRIES AND PUMPKIN SEEDS

116 GRAPE TRUFFLES AND TOFU SALTY WITH PISTACHIOS AND NUTS

117 CHICKPEAS FRUIT WITH HERBS AND CAULIFLOWER MAYONNAISE

118 NOODLES WITH SOY SAUCE

119 RAVIOLI STUFFED WITH POTATOES, BEANS, AND PESTO

120 CAULIFLOWER DUMPLINGS WITH CHLORINE

121 RISOTTO WITH CHOCOLATE AND ORANGE

122 LASAGNA WITH OLIVES SCAROLA AND WALNUTS

123 SCALA SEITAN
WITH MUSHROOMS

124 VEGETABLE GOULASH

126 SEITAN ROAST WITH
FRIARIELLI AND SUN DRIED
TOMATOES

127 VEGAN MEATBALLS WITH
PUMPKIN AND POTATOES
STUFFED WITH SPINACH

128 VEGAN CAKE FOR PARTY

129 CAKE WITH POTATO CREAM
CHOCOLATE DESSERT

130 SOFT CORN TACOS WITH
CAKES, POBLANOS, AND CORN

131 PERUVIAN GREEN SAUCE

132 ASPARAGUS IN VIENNA

133 ASPARAGUS WITH LEMON

172 PEASANT STYLE THIMBLES

173 POLENTA AND MUSHROOMS

174 MARINA POLENTA CAKE

175 CREPE TREVISO

176 SOFT PEN

177 PATIO PENS

178 SOFT PEN

179 PATIO PENS

180 BAKED TURKEY

INTRODUCTION

The One Meal A Day (OMAD) diet is an alternative to time-limited fasting, like traditional fasting. However, unlike intermittent fasting which generally allows for a four to eight hour stay, the OMAD diet has a one-hour window to eat. So it's fast during the other 23 hours of the day. Although various forms of intensive feeding have been recognized as an effective way of eating, nutritionists do not recommend the OMAD diet and it can be dangerous for people with health problems. This is what you need to know. OMAD is the longest form of fasting, aside from a 23: 1 fast (23 hours fast and 1 hour fast).

In its purest sense, OMAD is not
indicate a calorie restriction or specific
Macronutrient composition. That said, we
encourage you to continue with our
healthy and healthy diet at that meal.
And make sure you keep eating until the
end. for the other dishes of the OMAD diet
in addition. Meals on this diet can range
from a double burger
and french fries to a salad
richer in vegetables,
roasted vegetables, whole grains, beans,
nuts, and seeds. The idea is to limit
your calorie intake ou ou de
day, you can feast on meals
(usually referred to as a one hour
window) and lose weight again.
Waterfall
used and coffee are available, but for
the rest, the kitchen is closed all day.

WHAT IS THE OMAD DIET?

The **OMAD** diet or one meal a day is a
fasting method which, of course, consists
of eating only once a day. The
the one meal a day diet is a weight loss
program
where a person only eats one meal a day. On
this floor, they won't even be to the east.
drink something that contains calories
most of the day. It is a type of
intermittent fasting. It alternates for
a long time.
periods without eating or drinking
anything that contains calories with short
windows of time to eat. The diet that uses a
type of intermittent fasting
called 23: 1. This means a person
spends 23 hours a day fasting, leaving
only 1 hour a day to consume
calorie.

Most people who follow this diet eat
their food for dinner, therefore
Soon **still until night follows.**
However, some Research
suggests that having breakfast
can help control blood sugar
later in the day and reduce the risk of
type 2 diabetes. More research
contradicts these conclusions,
suggesting to skip breakfast
May **really be a strategy useful for**
some people in managing their total
calorie intake.

WHY OMAN
DIET WORKS

With thousands of trendy diets, it is becoming increasingly difficult to determine which is effective, which is safe, which is healthy and which is best suited to our individual needs. The nomadic diet is effective precisely because it is not another weight loss program, but rather a scientifically proven lifestyle weight management plan. Its principles are based on scientific studies that reveal what really works to lose weight and keep it off.

It also provides workable solutions to help those facing an extremely difficult or persistent weight loss problem. The Omad Diet tries to help you deal with the root cause of weight gain, which is a disrupted circadian rhythm. If you fix the cause of the problem, the problem will be fixed permanently. The elaborate diet provides simple and straightforward guidelines, making it easy to follow this plan for life and achieve lasting weight loss.

CAN YOU THINK OF EATING ONE MEAL A DAY?

When you only eat one meal a day, you are probably consuming far fewer calories than normal. A reduced calorie intake generally results in weight loss; Large-scale studies have found that people who fasted and people who limited their calorie intake in general lost the same amount of weight. It is very easy to feel deprived while practicing the OMAD diet, which could lead to binges and falling out of the car. Prolonged periods of restriction often result in weight cycles (ie, "yo-yo diets") and changes in hunger hormones and metabolism. Eventually, you may feel hungrier after trying the one meal a day diet than before starting this limited plan.

BONIATO GNOCCHI
WITH BROCCOLI

Preparation: 40 minutes
Cooking: 40 minutes
Total time: 1 hour and 20 min
For: 4 people
ingredients
600 g of sweet potatoes
(yam / American potatoes)
300 g of flour 0
500 g of broccoli
1 dry chilli
1 clove of garlic
salt
Extra virgin olive oil
Peeling tools
Rigagnocchi cream
Cooking!
Wash the potatoes well and, without
peeling them, cover them with water
in a saucepan and bring to a boil.
Cook until the potatoes are cooked in
lightly salted water: to be sure, prick
with a

fork, which must enter without encountering resistance. As soon as the potatoes are cooked, drain them and, while they are still hot, peel them and pass them to the food processor; then let them cool and season: if they are not tasty enough, add a pinch of salt. In the meantime, peel the broccoli and cut them into small pieces and steam them for 12 minutes, they must still be crunchy. We prepare the dough
Pour the flour into the bowl with the potatoes and knead until the mixture is smooth, not sticky but smooth. The quantities of flour are indicative, you may need more or less depending on the type of potatoes (more or less floury, more or less old, more or less watery). Form the gnocchi
Take part of the dough, flour a wooden cutting board and use it

with your hands form a roll with a
diameter of about 1-1.5 cm. Cut the roll
into 1 cm pieces. Flour the gnocchi
drain and pass each gnocchi on its
surface to print the characteristic lines
until the dough is finished. Place the
gnocchi on a well floured baking
sheet. cook the gnocchi
Put a large pot with plenty of salted water
on the stove and bring to the boil.
Meanwhile, in a pan, brown a clove of
garlic and a chili in a little extra virgin
olive oil. After a few minutes, add the
steamed broccoli and cook for a few
minutes, stirring constantly, and season
with salt.
As soon as the water boils, add a few
gnocchi at a time, and as soon as they
rise to the surface, remove them with a
slotted spoon and pour them into the
pan. When all the gnocchi are cooked,
sauté them for a minute with the sauce
and serve immediately while they are
still hot.

CANEDERLI WITH CHICORY AND SPINACH

Preparation: 30 min Cooking: 75 min
Total time: 1 hour 45 min
For: 4 people
ingredients
200 g of stale bread
60 g of fresh spinach
70 g of chicory
150 ml of vegetable broth
1 clove of garlic ½ shallot
2 teaspoons of chickpea flour
2 teaspoons of almond flour
2 teaspoons of flour 0
2 teaspoons of nutritional yeast
5 sage leaves
Breadcrumbs to taste
Salt and pepper for the broth.
1 onion 1 shallot 2 carrots
2 stalks of celery 1 courgette
Soy sauce 2.5 l of water
Utensils pots pans
non-stick bowls ¡A
to cook!
Let's start with the broth.
Thoroughly clean all the vegetables

broth. Cut the onion and shallot into 4 wedges, the carrots, celery and courgettes in half lengthwise and then each half into 3 large pieces. Pour the vegetables into a large pot and cover with water. Bring to a boil and simmer for at least an hour. Towards the end of cooking, add a few tablespoons of soy sauce (it will give flavor and color to the broth) and season with salt. Let it cool down. Cook the spinach and chicory, fry the garlic clove with a drizzle of oil in a pan. After a couple of minutes, add the spinach and season with salt and pepper. Cook just enough for them to dry and flavor. Remove from heat and set aside. In another pan, fry the chopped shallot with a drizzle of oil, the finely chopped sage,, and a pinch of salt. Prepare the meatballs Finely chop the stale bread (if you find it difficult to do it with your hands, use a serrated knife) and separate it into two different bowls (100g in each bowl). Pour 75 ml of hot broth into each bowl and start working the bread until the mixture is smooth. Then pour the spinach into one of the bowls with the bread and chicory in the other. Add to each mixture a teaspoon of chickpea flour, one of flour 0, one of almond flour and one of nutritional yeast, salt, and pepper. Mix the two compounds separately until you get a smooth and moldable dough with your hands. If necessary, add broth or breadcrumbs to adjust the consistency. Shape into balls slightly larger than a walnut and place them on a plate. You should finish with 6 radicchio gnocchi and 6 spinach gnocchi. And now the cooking: bring the vegetable broth back to the boil and gently dip the gnocchi into it.

THAI PADS

Preparation: 20 minutes
(+ 30 min soaking)
Cooking: 5 minutes
Total time: 25 minutes
For: 4 people
ingredients
320 g of rice noodles
200 g of tofu
140 g of carrots
200 g of broccoli
130 g of mushrooms
60 g of bean sprouts
1 spring onion
1 lime
50 g of natural peanut
sesame oil for the
dressing
3 spoons of soy sauce
2 spoons of sesame oil
1 spoon of tamarind paste

1 tablespoon of brown sugar
2 tsp molasses (or malt)
½ teaspoon of ground
ginger 120 g of water Tools
cooking
in the
wok.

First, soak the rice noodles in plenty of water at room temperature for 30 minutes and let them soften. In the meantime, cut the tofu into cubes, chop the white part of the spring onion, effloresce the broccoli, cut the carrots into sticks and slice the mushrooms. Separately, chop the peanuts into large pieces and set aside. Fry the tofu and vegetables. Heat a drizzle of sesame oil in a wok and saute the chopped tofu and chives for a couple of minutes over medium-high heat until golden brown. Remove from the wok and reserve.

Heat a little more oil
sesame and this time brown the
broccoli together
with carrots and mushrooms
until golden brown but still
crunchy, then remove the vegetables
also the wok. Season the noodles
Pour in all the sauce ingredients
the pan, heat and add the noodles
drained from the soaking water. Cook them
for a minute, then add the tofu,
sauteed vegetables, and bean sprouts e
fry over high heat for another minute
to flavor everything. Serve the noodles,
garnish each dish with peanuts ea
freshly squeezed lime wedge when
be ready to eat. Finally decorate
with the green part of the chopped chives
in the circles.

WHOLEMEAL PASTA WITH LETTUCE PESTO

Preparation: 5 minutes
Cooking: 10 minutes
Total time: 15 minutes
For 6 people

ingredients
500 g of wholemeal pasta
230 g of clean lettuce
100 g of extra virgin olive oil
40 g of walnuts
30 g of pine nuts + 2 tablespoons
for decoration
1 ½ tablespoon of nutritional yeast
½ clove of garlic
Salt and pepper
Tools Hand
blender

Cooking!,
Let's prepare the lettuce pesto
Wash, peel, and slice the lettuce. Pour
the oil, walnuts, pine nuts, nutritional
yeast, garlic, part of the lettuce, salt and
pepper into the tall glass of the hand
mixer. Start beating with the mixer until
creamy and add more lettuce when the
level in the glass has dropped. Once the
lettuce is ready, blend until smooth and
homogeneous. Season the pasta
Cook the pasta in abundant salted water
and drain it al dente, reserving a glass of
cooking water. Season the pasta with the
lettuce pesto, diluting with a little water if
it is too thick. Toast the pine nuts in a hot
skillet until golden brown. Serve the pasta,
decorate each portion with pine nuts and
serve.

WHOLEMEAL BUTTERFLIES WITH ONION AND GREEN OLIVES

Preparation: 10 minutes
Cooking: 10 minutes
Total time: 20 minutes
For: 4 people

ingredients
320 g of whole butterflies
150 g of green olives
20 g of salted capers
1 Tropea onion
1 sprig of rosemary
chili powder
1 clove of garlic
extra virgin olive oil to taste

Cooking!
First, finely chop the green olives and
wash the capers under running water to
remove excess salt. Heat a drizzle of extra
virgin olive oil in a non-stick pan
and add the clove of garlic, chili,
rosemary and then the capers
and green olives. Let it cook for
a few minutes and then remove
the garlic. cook the pasta
Cook the pasta in abundant salted
water then drain it al dente and finish
cooking in a pan with olives and
capers for seasoning. Finely chop the
onion and add it raw to the pasta.
Enjoy your meal!

UDON WITH SAUCE PEANUTS AND SESAME

Preparation: 5 minutes
Cooking time: 10 min
Total time: 15 minutes
For: 4 people

ingredients
350g udon (Japanese noodles)
50 g of peanut butter
3 tablespoons of soy sauce
1 tablespoon of sesame seeds
1 tablespoon of sesame oil
1 teaspoon of Sriracha
(Thai hot sauce)
½ a teaspoon of ground ginger
½ a teaspoon of garlic inside
powder 100 ml of broth
vegetables
1 spring onion
Peanuts al
taste

Cooking!
Let's prepare the peanut sauce.
In a small saucepan, add the peanut
butter, soy sauce, sesame oil, vegetable
stock, ginger, garlic and sriracha and
simmer for a few minutes until smooth
and homogeneous. . Let's move on to
the don. Boil the udon in boiling salted
water, drain, and rinse with cold water.
Pour them into a bowl or put them
back in the pot and mix them with the
peanut sauce. Serve to garnish each
plate with sesame seeds, a few peanuts,
and the green part of the chives cut into
rings.

SOFT PASTA AND CHICKPEAS

Preparation: 20 minutes
Cooking: 70 minutes
Total time: 1 hour and 30 min
For: 4 people
ingredients
120 g of dried chickpeas
150 g of small wholemeal pasta
1 onion
1 carrot
1 celery
1 clove of garlic
1 Pope
1 spoon of tomato
paste with sage
Pottage
Rosemary
1 piece of kombu seaweed
2 bay leaves
Salt and pepper

Cooking.
We cook the chickpeas
Rinse the chickpeas and soak them in plenty of water overnight. Drain them, pour them into a pressure cooker, cover them with cold water and add the bay leaves and the piece of kombu seaweed. Close the pressure cooker and put it on the stove. Cook the chickpeas for 40 minutes after the pot starts whistling. If you don't have a pressure cooker, hyperbole for at least an hour and a half. Prepare the sauté. Finely chop a sprig of rosemary and a few sage leaves. Heat a drizzle of extra virgin olive oil in a large pot and sauté the aromatic herbs and the garlic clove for a couple of minutes. Peel and chop the onion, carrot and celery and add them to the pot, along with a pinch of salt.

Fry everything for 5 minutes. Also add the chopped potato and tomato paste and cook for a few minutes.

Add the rest of the ingredients, add the chickpeas drained from the cooking water, a pinch of salt and pepper, cover with the vegetable broth and bring to a boil. Cook for 10 minutes, until the potatoes, begin to soften. Add the pasta and cook for the time indicated on the package. Look at the amount of water you have in the pot, it should be enough to cook the pasta and leave a soft and warm bottom, but not liquid like a soup. Serve hot immediately.

SPAGHETTI OF SPELLED WITH LEEK AND SAFFRON CREAM OF CHICKPEAS

Preparation: 10 minutes
Cooking time: 20 min
Total time: 30 minutes
For: 4 people

ingredients
360 g of whole spelled spaghetti
260 g of cooked chickpeas
1 leek
160 g of unsweetened soy milk
1 sachet of saffron
1 tablespoon of chopped sage
Salt and pepper
food processor tools

We cook!

Let's prepare the chickpea cream. Combine the chickpeas, soy milk, saffron, a pinch of salt and a pinch of pepper in the food processor and blend until smooth and creamy. Cook the leeks. Finely chop the sage and brown it lightly in a large pan with a little extra virgin olive oil for a minute. Clean and wash the leeks well, then cut them lengthwise into strips about 20 cm long and half a centimeter wide. Sauté them in a pan with the sage for 10 minutes until tender, season with salt and pepper. Season the pasta

Cook the pasta in abundant salted water, after listening to it, reserving a glass of water. Fry the spaghetti together with the leek and chickpea cream, adding a little of the pasta cooking water until a homogeneous sauce is obtained. Serve hot immediately.

WHOLEMEAL PASTA WITH ARTICHOKES

Preparation: 15 minutes
Cooking: 25 min
Total time: 40 minutes
For: 4 people
ingredients
350 wholemeal pasta
6 artichokes
2 cloves of garlic
1 ½ tablespoon of chopped parsley
Extra virgin olive oil Salt e
pepper
Cooking!
We clean the artichokes
Eliminate the hardest outer leaves of
each artichoke, then cut the top to
remove the terminal part of the leaves
that are stringy. Clean the stem well
with a sharp knife. Open the artichoke
in half and remove the internal tip, then
cut it into wedges.

If you don't cook them immediately, soak the artichokes in a bowl with cold water and lemon to prevent them from turning black. It is also advisable to carry out these cleaning operations with gloves, to avoid blackening hands and nails. Frying the artichokes Cut the two garlic cloves in half lengthwise and fry them in a large pan with a drizzle of extra virgin olive oil until golden brown. Add the artichokes, drained of water, and, if necessary, the lemon and cook for 15 minutes, until soft and slightly golden. Season with salt and pepper, add the parsley, and remove the garlic. Season the pasta. Boil the pasta in abundant salted water and drain it al dente, reserving a glass of water. Brown the pasta with the artichokes for a minute, adding, if necessary, a little pasta cooking water. Once well flavored,

FENNEL TAGLIOLINI WITH LEMON AND TEMPEH CRUMBLE

Preparation: 15 minutes
Cooking: 10 minutes
Total time: 25 minutes
For: 4 people
ingredients
350 g of noodles
2 large fennel
150 g of tempera
2 teaspoons of curry
1 large clove of garlic
1 lemon Salt
taste
virgin olive oil
extra cooking.
Start by cleaning the fennel, then cut it into 4 wedges and slice it thinly in the direction of the grain.

Meanwhile, put a drizzle of extra virgin olive oil and 1 clove of garlic cut in half in a non-stick pan and brown. Before adding the fennel, put 2 teaspoons of curry powder in a pan and let it dissolve in the oil. Add the fennel, season with salt and sauté for about ten minutes over medium heat until just tender, then half cooked, sprinkle with lemon juice. In another pan, with a drizzle of oil, crumble the tempeh into small crumbs, season with salt and brown over high heat until golden brown, creating a light crust. At this point all that remains is to cook the tagliatelle in abundant salted water. The advice is to drain the pasta a minute before finishing and season it with the fennel so that it is well seasoned,

FUSILLI TOMATOES
DRIED CASHEWS

Preparation: 10 minutes
Cooking: 15 min
Total time: 25 minutes
For: 4 people

ingredients
320 g of fusilli
half a red onion
40 g of natural cashews
6 dried tomatoes without oil
chili powder to taste
Extra virgin olive oil al
to taste Salt to taste
Lemon juice to taste
Cooking!
We cut the tomatoes
First, soak the dried tomatoes in
hot water: this will allow them to do
so
hydrate still;

When they are soft, first cut them lengthwise and then widthwise to obtain rectangular slices that are not too large. Now it's time to cut the onion into thin slices.

In a non-stick pan, put oil, onion, a pinch of salt and red pepper and fry over medium heat for a few minutes until the onion is tender and transparent. In the pan add the cashews (if you prefer you can also chop them coarsely with a knife) and the wet dried tomatoes. Season the pasta Now proceed to boil the pasta, taking care to finish cooking one minute earlier than indicated. Drain the pasta and pour it directly into the pan with the sauce: add a pinch of salt, brown over high heat, and, finally, add a little lemon juice if you want. Serve and enjoy your food!

FETTUCCINE EDAMAME WITH PUMPKIN, LENTILS AND WALNUTS

Preparation: 10 minutes

Cooking time: 35 min

Total time: 45 minutes

For: 4 people

ingredients

350 g edamame fettuccine

400 g of clean pumpkin

80 g of dried lentils

40 g of walnuts

½ onion 1

bay leaf

sage

Salt and pepper

Let's cook! Let's prepare the sauce.

Rinse the lentils well under running water, pour them into a saucepan, cover them with cold water, add the bay leaf and bring to a boil.

Boil ththe e lentils for about twenty minutes, or until they are soft but not mushy. Drain, remove the bay leaf and set it aside. Finely chop the onion and sage and brown in a pan with a drizzle of oil and a pinch of salt. Add the lentils and the minced pumpkin and cook for about ten minutes until they are cooked but keeping the shape. Season with salt and pepper. Let's cook the edamame fettuccine. Boil the edamame fettuccine in abundant salted water for the time indicated on the package. Listen to them, reserving a cup of cooking water. Brown the pasta in a pan with the sauce, garnish with coarsely chopped walnuts, a drizzle of oil, and enough water to obtain a not too dry sauce. Serve immediately.

PENNE WITH SOY SAUCE AND SAFFRON CREAM

Preparation: 25 minutes
Cooking: 50 minutes
Total time: 1 hour 15 min
For: 4 people
ingredients
320 g of wholemeal penne rigate
150 soybean granules
2 medium carrots
1 stalk of celery
1 onion
1 sprig of sage
100 ml of white wine
1 clove of garlic
1 teaspoon granulated vegetable
broth For the sauce
2 tablespoons of nutritional yeast
200 g of soy cream or other
vegetable bread (rice or
oatmeal)

1 sachet of saffron
A pinch of nutmeg
processor tools
food without pan
We cook!
First, prepare the ragù: soak the soya granules in warm water for about twenty minutes; drain and reserve.
After cleaning the carrots and celery, cut them into large pieces and put them in a food processor together with the onion - chop everything very finely. In a large pan with a drizzle of extra virgin olive oil, fry the garlic until golden brown, add the carrot, celery, and onion and simmer for a couple of minutes. Cook the meat sauce. At this point, add the soy grains and sage leaves to the stir-fried meat sauce.

Over high heat, cook all the ingredients for about ten minutes. Now add the wine and let everything evaporate. Dissolve the vegetable broth in half a glass of warm water, add it to the sauce and cover with a lid: let it cook for about 40 minutes over low heat. Let's prepare the sauce. In the meantime, put the cream, saffron, nutritional yeast,and nutmeg in a saucepan over the heat: bring to the boil and, stirring constantly, cook for about 5 minutes so that the powders melt perfectly. Finally, before serving, cook the pasta in abundant salted water: season with the cream and the meat sauce.

WHOLE SPAGHETTI WITH CHICKPEAS AND PLUMS

Preparation: 10 minutes
Cooking: 10 minutes
Total time: 20 minutes
For: 4 people

ingredients
320 g of wholemeal spaghetti
200 g of cooked chickpeas
30 gr of black olives
16 plums
2 tomatoes salt
taste
extra virgin olive oil
black pepper to taste
taste

Cooking!
Wash the cherry tomatoes, cut them in half, and remove the internal seeds. Cut them into cubes and put them in a large bowl. Separately, coarsely chop the black olives and dried figs. Add the chopped cherry tomatoes to the bowl. cook the pasta

Cook the pasta in abundant salted water and drain it al dente. Pour the spaghetti into the bowl with the chopped vegetables and prunes. Add the cooked chickpeas and season with extra virgin olive oil and salt if necessary. Add a pinch of black pepper and mix to mix all ingredients well.

WHOLE SPAGHETTI WITH AUBERGINES, WALNUT FLUSH AND BLACK OLIVES

Preparation: 10 minutes
Cooking: 20 minutes
Total time: 30 minutes
For 2 people
ingredients
180 g of wholemeal spaghetti
15 cherry tomatoes
20 g of pitted black olives
1 large eggplant
1 clove of garlic
Extra virgin olive oil
nutmeg to taste
Salt to taste
Cooking!
Peel and cut the aubergine into
cubes and leave it to marinate for
a few minutes in hot water and
salt to remove the bitter taste that
characterizes this vegetable.

After having drained the aubergines from the water, which in the meantime has darkened, brown a clove of garlic in a non-stick pan with a drizzle of extra virgin olive oil; When the oil is golden brown, remove it from the pan and add the chopped aubergines. Season with salt and add the fresh nutmeg: we recommend grating the whole nutmeg because it releases its aroma better. Add the other ingredients, Peel, and cut the tomatoes and olives into wedges, add them to the aubergines, and continue cooking until the vegetables are soft. Cook the pasta and serve. Cook the pasta in abundant salted water, leaving it al dente, and finish cooking in a pan with the vegetables.

WHOLE PASTA WITH PUMPKIN SPICE

Preparation: 60 minutes
Cooking: 20 minutes
Total time: 1 hour and 20 min
For: 4 people
ingredients
320 g of short wholemeal pasta
4 courgettes 60 g of apple cider vinegar
30 g of water extra virgin olive
oil for frying 1 clove of garlic
pepper and salt fresh thyme to
decorate Mandolin Kitchen
utensils!
Wash the courgettes under running
water to remove any residual dirt, then,
with the help of a mandolin, cut them
into slices a few millimeters thick.
Sprinkle them with salt and let them
rest for at least an hour so that they lose
part of the water of their vegetation.
After this time, rinse quickly under
running water,

Dry them with kitchen paper and then fry them in abundant extra virgin olive oil until golden brown. Drain the courgettes and remove the excess oil with kitchen paper, then place them in a bowl and season with pepper and, if necessary, a little salt. Add the apple cider vinegar In a small saucepan, bring the apple cider vinegar to a boil along with the water and coarsely chopped garlic. Season the zucchini with the vinegar mixture and marinate for as long as possible (up to 24 hours) so that the vegetables take on a good flavor. Cook the pasta. Bring the salted water to a boil in a saucepan. Cook the pasta for the necessary time, drain and season with the zucchini shoulder blade and a few leaves of fresh thyme. Lemon thyme will be perfect, a particular variety of thyme whose seedlings are sometimes found in specialized nurseries; "classic"

POTATO GNOCCHI
WITH FLOUR
PEAS AND BASIL

Preparation: 30 minutes
Cooking: 3 minutes
Total time: 33 minutes
For: 4 people
ingredients
100 g of pea flour
100 g of wholemeal spelled flour
110 ml of water
20 g of potato starch
5 g of salt
3 basil leaves
2 potatoes inside
the kitchen!
Boil the potatoes in plenty of water
and then let them cool, peel them,
and cut them into cubes.

In a large bowl, sift the pea flour, the wholemeal spelled flour, and the potato starch. Stir to mix the ingredients well, then add the salt and water little by little. Knead

the dough until a smooth and

homogeneous dough is obtained,

depending on the

the flour used may need to add a little

more

Waterfall.

gnocchi

Make long sticks with the dough and cut them into pieces of about 2 cm. Roll each of these onto the wooden board, pressing gently with the thumb of your hand or the tines of a fork and sliding to the opposite end. When you have finished with all the batter, cook the gnocchi in abundant salted water for about 3 minutes, then listen to them and sauté them in a pan with a drizzle of extra virgin olive oil, basil, and diced boiled potatoes. Serve immediately still hot.

TAGLIATELLE WITH CARROT AND BASIL SAUCE

Preparation: 10 minutes
Cooking time: 20 min
For: 4 people
ingredients
500 g of tomato puree
320 g of wholemeal noodles
4 carrots 1 onion
extra virgin olive oil with basil salt to taste Cook!
Finely chop the onion, then heat a drizzle of extra virgin olive oil in a non-stick pan and quickly brown the onion. Add the diced carrots and cook for about 5 minutes, allowing them to flavor. Add the tomato sauce
Pour in the tomato puree, season with salt and pepper and cook for about 15 minutes or until the carrots are just softened. Cook the wholemeal tagliatelle in plenty of salted water and once drained, season them with the carrot sauce and decorate with a few basil leaves.

TAGLIATELLE WITH PESTO ARUGULA AND CASHEW

Preparation: 10 min Cooking: 6 min
Total time: 16 min to 4
people Ingredients
320 g of wholemeal noodles
110 g of rocket 100 g of cashews
salt to taste Delicate extra virgin
olive oil You're cooking!
In a tall, narrow glass, add the rocket
leaves followed by the cashews and a
pinch of salt. Work the ingredients with
the blades of a mixer and add the extra
virgin olive oil until a homogeneous
cream without lumps is obtained. Cook
the noodles Separately, cook the noodles
in abundant salted water for the time
necessary to cook them al dente. In the
end, drain and pour into a large bowl.
Season with two tablespoons of rocket
cream and, if necessary, season with salt.
Serve the noodles hot or warm.

SPAGHETTI WITH SADDLE WITH RIBS AND DRIED TOMATOES

Preparation: 15 min Cooking: 25 min
Total time: 40 min for 4
people Ingredients
350 g of buckwheat spaghetti
1 bunch of ribs (about 500 g)
3-4 dried tomatoes
2 tablespoons of capers
1 clove of garlic
1 teaspoon of oregano
1 teaspoon of thyme
4 tablespoons of breadcrumbs
wholemeal for cooking!
We cook the ribs
Wash and clean the ribs, thin the stems
by cutting them in 3 lengthwise and
dividing them into pieces of 5-6 cm
together with the leaves. Blanch the
stems in lightly salted boiling water for 5
minutes, then add the leaves and
continue cooking for another 5 minutes.
Drain the vegetables and set them aside.

Prepare the pasta sauce
Heat a drizzle of oil in a large pan with the peeled garlic clove, thyme and oregano, keeping the heat low so that the aromatic herbs impregnate the oil with their aroma. Rinse the capers and chop them coarsely together with the dried tomatoes, then add them to the pan with 2-3 tablespoons of dried tomato preservation oil. Sauté for a few minutes, then add the ribs to the pan and sauté for 7-8 minutes to flavor. Season with salt. Boil the pasta and serve. Mix the breadcrumbs with two tablespoons of oil and toast it in a small pan until golden brown. Meanwhile, boil the spaghetti in abundant salted water, leaving them al dente. Drain them and add them to the sauce together with half a ladle of their cooking water.

WHOLE PASTA WITH CHESTNUT AND HAZELNUTS BEACH SAUCE

Preparation: 5 minutes
Cooking: 15 min
Total time: 20 minutes
For: 4 people

ingredients
320 g of wholemeal pasta
100 g of chestnut flour
hot vegetable broth (about 500 ml)
80 g of extra virgin olive oil
Rosemary
hazelnuts to taste
salt

Cooking!

Chestnut bechamel Finely chop the rosemary. Meanwhile, heat the extra virgin olive oil with the chestnut flour in a saucepan. As soon as the mixture reaches a boil, add the vegetable broth, always stirring with a few sticks to avoid the formation of lumps and until the desired creaminess is reached. Add the rosemary and season with salt. Wholemeal pasta Cook the pasta in abundant salted water. Meanwhile, toast the hazelnuts in a non-stick pan, being careful not to burn them. At the end let them cool and then chop them coarsely. Drain the pasta and dress it with the chestnut sauce and the chopped toasted hazelnuts.

COLD PASTA OF FAST AND CREAMY VEGETABLES

Preparation: 10 minutes
Total time: 10 minutes
For: 4 people
ingredients
320 g of wholemeal fusilli
3 carrots 2 courgettes
20 cherry or cherry tomatoes
160 g of boiled sweet corn
200 g of cooked pinto beans
2 tablespoons of chia seeds
40 g of unsweetened soy yogurt
turmeric to taste salt to taste
extra virgin olive oil
Cooking!
Vegetables
Clean, peel and chop the carrots. Cut the cherry tomatoes and courgettes in the same way, then add the sweet corn and borlotti beans.

Season the vegetables with extra
virgin olive oil, olive oil, and a pinch
of salt. Add the chia seeds and mix
to combine all the ingredients Pasta
Cook the pasta in abundant salted water,
drain it al dente, and immediately put it
under cold water, stirring constantly
with your hands. adding a drizzle of oil,
until
complete cold. The cream
In a small bowl, mix the vegetable
yogurt with turmeric to make the
cream softer and more colorful. Then
add a pinch of salt. Season the pasta
with chopped vegetables. Serve the
pasta decorated with turmeric cream.

MALTAGLIATI WITH CHESTNUTS WITH PUMPKIN RAGU

ingredients
For the maltagliati
200 g of semolina flour
50 g of chestnut flour
155 ml of water 5 g of salt
for the seasoning
300 g of pumpkin
8 shiitake mushrooms
extra virgin olive oil 1/2 onion
Cooking!
Preparations
First, soak the shiitake mushrooms. Separately, sift the flours in a bowl so that there are no lumps. Add the salt and then slowly add the water, working the ingredients with your hands until the mixture is smooth and elastic. Form a ball and let it rest at room temperature, wrapped in cling film, for at least 30 minutes. Maltagliati After resting, roll out the dough a

on a pastry board, sprinkle with a thin layer of flour and try to reach a thickness of 3 millimeters. With a knife, form rectangular strips 2 inches wide and obtain from the dough some very irregular rhombuses that you will place on a floured surface. Dice the onion and brown it in a non-stick pan with a drizzle of extra virgin olive oil. As soon as the onion has taken a little color, add the shiitake, which you have squeezed and diced in the meantime; continue cooking for about 10 minutes. Grate the pumpkin or cut it into very small cubes and add it to the pan with the onion and mushrooms. Cook quickly over high heat for about 5 minutes and, if necessary, add a ladle of hot water.

WHOLE SHELL WITH EDAMAME

Preparation: 5 minutes
Cooking: 15 min
Total time: 20 minutes
For: 4 people

ingredients
300 g of frozen edamame
120g canned peas, drained
320 g of whole shells
Lemon peel
4 basil leaves
extra virgin olive oil
salt

We cook!
Boil the soybeans
Pour the frozen edamame beans
directly into the water and hyperbola
for 5 minutes. In a non-stick pan, heat
a drizzle of extra virgin olive oil and
quickly brown the drained peas. After a
few minutes, add the edamame and
season with salt. Add the lemon zest
and basil and cook for two minutes
over high heat.
Cook the pasta and serve.
Also boil the shells in abundant salted
water. Scrupolle al dente and mix them
with the legumes, taking care to mix all
the ingredients well. Serve garnished
with fresh basil.

PLEUROTUS MUSHROOMS GRATINATE

Preparation: 15 minutes
 Cooking: 30 minutes
Total time: 45 minutes
 For: 4 people

ingredients
500 g of Pleurotus mushrooms
5 tablespoons of breadcrumbs
 spoons of olive oil
 extra virgin
olive oil
kilos
Instruments
Baking tray Silicone baking mat

Cooking!
First, clean the mushrooms very
well, removing the earthy parts.

Then line the pan with the silicone pan, brush with a drizzle of oil to which you have added a pinch of red pepper and arrange the mushrooms in a single layer. Season the breadcrumbs with two tablespoons of oil and a pinch of red pepper. Salt the mushrooms and then cover them with breadcrumbs. Bake them in a static oven at 180 ° C for 30 minutes, increasing the temperature to 200 ° C in the last 5 minutes of cooking to brown the gratin. Serve your mushrooms au gratin piping hot as a garnish.

ROASTED RED POTATOES WITH HERBS AND CORN

Preparation: 10 min Cooking time:
20 min Total time: 30 min Stop
4 people Ingredients
500 g of red potatoes
1 teaspoon of rosemary, chopped
1 teaspoon of chopped sage
1 teaspoon of oregano
2 tablespoons of cornstarch
salt and oil
Cooking.
Wash the potatoes very well and cut
them into wedges without removing the
skin. In a bowl season them with a nice
pinch of salt, cornflour, rosemary, sage,
and oregano, and finish with a drizzle of
extra virgin olive oil. Transfer the
seasoned potatoes to a fairly large pan
and spread them out in a single layer.
Bake in a static oven at 200 ° C for 20
minutes until soft and golden.

FENNELS WITH TURMERIC WITH POTATOES AND ONIONS

Preparation: 10 minutes
Cooking time: 20 min
Total time: 30 minutes
For: 4 people

ingredients

2 fennel
1 onion
2 Potato
1 ½ teaspoon of turmeric
1 teaspoon of oregano
¼ teaspoon of ground ginger ¼ teaspoon of garam masala Salt and pepper

Cooking.

Using a sharp knife, cut the onion and fennel and cut the potatoes into cubes separately after peeling them. In a saucepan, fry the turmeric, garam masala, ginger and oregano in a little oil and add the onions, letting them cook for 5 minutes with a pinch of salt. Then add the potatoes and brown for another 5 minutes.

Finally, pour the fennel into the pot and continue cooking for another 10-15 minutes with a lid on until the vegetables are soft and cooked. Serve immediately hot as an accompaniment to the main course or as a sauce for pasta.

FENNEL PIZZAIOLA

Preparation: 10 minutes
Cooking: 25 min
Total time: 35 minutes
For: 4 people

ingredients

2 fennel
200 g of cherry tomatoes
150 g of tomato sauce
1 tablespoon of capers
60 g of olives
1 clove of garlic
A few leaves of fresh basil

Cooking!

Fry the garlic clove in a non-stick pan and in the meantime slice the not too thin fennel. Put in a pan, season with salt and brown for a couple of minutes to flavor. At this point cover with a lid and cook for 15 minutes. Season the fennel Coarsely chop the capers and cut into cubes

sliced olives. add the tomato puree,
olives, capers, and fennel and
continue cooking for the others
5 minute
s. To
serve
Finally, add the halved cherry tomatoes
and cook for another 5 minutes or until
the cherry tomatoes begin to soften.
Top with a few fresh basil leaves and
serve immediately.

WINTER VEGETABLES BAKED WITH 4-FLAVORED SAUCE

Preparation: 15 minutes
Cooking: 35 minutes
Total time: 50 minutes
For: 4-6 people
ingredients
200 g of broccoli florets
200 g of cauliflower flowers
200 g of red potatoes
200 g of pumpkin
200 g of Brussels sprouts
1 teaspoon of rosemary
1 teaspoon of oregano
Salt and pepper
For the 4 flavor sauce
1 tablespoon of soy sauce
1 tablespoon of lemon juice
1 tablespoon of mustard
1 tablespoon of rice malt
Instruments
Baking tray
Silicone tray

Cooking!
Start by washing all the vegetables well, then butter the broccoli and cauliflower, cut the Brussels sprouts in half and dice the red potatoes and squash.

cook the vegetables
Season the vegetables in a bowl with salt, oil, oregano and rosemary, place them on a baking tray, and bake in a preheated static oven at 180 ° C for 35-40 minutes until the vegetables are cooked.

We prepare the 4 flavors of the sauce. Meanwhile, in a bowl, mix the mustard with the soy sauce, lemon juice, and rice malt to create your 4-flavor sauce. Once the vegetables have been removed from the oven, sprinkle them with the sauce and serve hot or lukewarm.

BAKED ISABELLA PASTA

Preparation time: 1 hour and 15 '
 Cooking time: 20'

INGREDIENTS for four people: 400 g
giant penne 120 g butter 500 g
bechamel with breadcrumbs 300 g
frozen peas nutmeg 200 g mushrooms
pepper 250 g cooked ham salt 150 g
mozzarella Cook the peas in 50 g of butter
and the mushrooms separately, again in 50 g
of butter. Boil the penne a lot
al dente in salted water, drain and season
with bechamel, cooked ham
Cut the mozzarella into strips, the peas
and the mushrooms, add a pinch of
nutmeg,,, and arrange the pasta in a
greased pan with butter. Sprinkle the
surface with breadcrumbs and a few
drops of butter, then bake in a
preheated oven at 200 ° for 20 minutes.

SICILIAN CAKE

Preparation time: 1 hour and 15 minutes
Cooking time: 20 minutes
INGREDIENTS for four people: 400 g of
simple penne 200 g of mozzarella 3
aubergines oil 800 g of tomato pulp butter 2
shallots salt a bunch of basil pepper 150 g
of ricotta salt Cut the aubergines into thin
slices, add salt and let them lose the liquid
of vegetation on an inclined plane.
Meanwhile, chop the shallots, fry them in
four tablespoons of oil and add the tomato
pulp, basil, season and cook the sauce for
about 30 minutes over low heat. Cook the
penne al dente in salted water, season with
the tomato sauce, grease a pan, and
alternate layers of pasta, aubergines, and
slices of mozzarella until all the ingredients
are used up. Complete with a layer of
eggplant,

TUSCAN RAVIOLI

Preparation time: 1 hour and 30 minutes minutes Cooking time: 10 minutes

INGREDIENTS for four people: 400 g of egg pasta 2 cloves of garlic 300 g of dried beans 200 g of ricotta 200 g of olive oil 1 red pepper salt 1 yellow sage Soak the beans overnight, drain, put them in a saucepan with cold water, a tablespoon of oil, sage, rosemary and 1 clove of garlic and simmer for an hour and a half. Drain the cannellini beans, mash them and let them cool. Add the boiled cannellini beans to the ricotta and mix, adding rosemary, salt, pepper, and two tablespoons of oil. Roll out the dough and form strips: in the center spread the mixture of beans into piles, separated from each other, and with the remaining strips cover them, pressing with your fingers, and cut the rectangular ravioli. Peel the peppers, cut the stems into cubes and cook them in a saucepan with three tablespoons of oil and 1 clove of garlic. Pour the sauce over the ravioli cooked al dente, add a pinch of pepper and serve.

CANADIAN OAT COOKIES

ingredients

for 4 people 1 kg of oats 200 g of sugar 1 cup
of oil 1/2 cup of maple syrup a bag of yeast
or 50 g of brewer's yeast On a cutting board
mix the sugar and oats to form a source ,
add the oil and knead the dough with your
hands, making sure it is a little soft. Just
heat the maple syrup and add the yeast,
making it dissolve well. Add to the dough,
then let it rise for about ten minutes. With
your hands greased with grease, form balls
that we will then crush on the previously
greased mold (but I recommend you use
baking paper, which is more convenient).
Bake for half an hour at 180 ° C in a
preheated oven.

IRISH OAT DONUT

ingredients

for 4 people 350 g of oats 25 g of yeast 4 whole eggs a pinch of salt 100 g of butter 150 g of vanilla sugar 1 beaten egg granulated sugar Put 250 g of oats and yeast in a bowl. Spread the yeast with your hands, add the eggs and a pinch of salt, and start kneading, gradually incorporating the flour. Then add the hot butter and sugar, making the mixture absorb all the ingredients, and finally the vanilla. Work the dough vigorously, which is well melted, so that it acquires elasticity, and when it is evaluated, cover it with a cloth and let it rise for about 4 hours, until it has doubled its volume.

When the dough has risen, deflate it, beating it by hand, turning it on the table, and adding the rest of the flour little by little, if necessary bring it to the consistency of a very soft bread dough. Re-knead the dough vigorously and then give it the shape of a very large doña, which you place in a mold of about a foot in diameter, with low edges, and let it rise again until it has increased in volume and is smooth to the touch. . . the touch. It will take 3-4 hours. Once the dough has risen well, spread a very lightly beaten egg on the donut and sprinkle it with plenty of icing sugar. Bake in a preheated oven at 180 ° C for a good half hour. Remove the donut from the oven and leave it to cool on a baking sheet.

SWEET CREAM WITH OAT FRUITS

ingredients

for 4 people

100 g of oat flakes 1/2 liter of milk a package of sweet cream 100 g of strawberries 100 g of blueberries 100 g of blackberries 100 g of raspberries 4 tablespoons of sugar Crush the red berries in a blender and add to the cream. Bring the milk and sugar to a boil and pour in the oats, cook for 20 minutes, remove from the heat and allow to cool. Add the berries. Arrange the sweet cream in dessert bowls and let it cool in the fridge for a couple of hours before serving.

OATMEAL SWEET CREAM ORANGE

Ingredients

for 4 people

100 g of oat flakes 1/2 liter of milk a pack of cream for desserts 4 oranges 1 glass of Cointreau 4 tablespoons of sugar With a potato peeler, peel the oranges and cut the peel into julienne strips, taking care not to leave the white part, which can be bitter. Mash the orange pulp in a blender and add it to the cream. Bring the milk with the sugar and Cointreau to the boil and pour in the oats, cook for 20 minutes, remove from the heat and allow to cool. Add the pulp of the oranges. Arrange the sweet cream in dessert bowls, decorated with the stringy skin, and refrigerate for a couple of hours before serving.

SWEET OAT FLOUR
CREAM WITH CHESTNUTS

ingredients

for 4 people
100 g of oat flakes 1/2 liter of milk a
package of sweet cream 300 g of boiled
chestnuts 4 tablespoons of sugar Carefully
peel the chestnuts and mash the pulp with
a fork, then add them to the cream. Bring
the milk and sugar to a boil and pour in the
oats, cook for 20 minutes, then remove
from heat and allow to cool. Add the
chestnut pulp. Arrange the sweet cream in
dessert bowls and let it cool in the fridge
for a couple of hours before serving. If
crumbled iced brown is used instead of
chestnuts, the dessert is much tastier.

SWEET OAT CREAM
WITH STRAWBERRY GRAPES

ingredients
for 4 people
100 g of oat flakes 1/2 liter of milk a
package of cream for desserts 300 g of
strawberry grapes 1 glass of strawberry
wine 4 tablespoons of sugar Crush the
strawberry grapes with the peel, but after
removing the seeds, and mix it with the
cream. Bring the milk to a boil, to which
we added the strawberries with sugar,
and pour the oats, cook for 20 minutes,
remove from the heat and allow to cool.
Add the strawberry and grape cream.
Arrange the sweet cream in dessert bowls
and let it cool in the fridge for a couple of
hours before serving.

SWEET OAT CREAM WITH APPLES AND PINIONS

ingredients
for 4 people

100 g of oat flakes 1/2 liter of milk a
pack of cream for desserts 2 apples
100 g of pine nuts 4 tablespoons of sugar
Cut the apples into very thin slices, after
having peeled them, and chop the pine
nuts, then mix everything with the cream.
Bring the milk and sugar to a boil and
pour in the oats, simmering for 20
minutes. Then remove from heat and let
cool. Add the apple and pine nut mixture.
Arrange the sweet cream in dessert bowls
and let it cool in the fridge for a couple of
hours before serving.

SCOTTISH STYLE
SWEET OAT CREAM

ingredients

for 4 people

100 g of rolled oats 1/2 liter of milk 2 apples 2 pears 4 tablespoons of honey 50 g of walnuts A pinch of cinnamon Peel the apples and pears and chop them coarsely together with the walnuts. Bring the milk to a boil and pour in the oats, stirring. Add the honey and cinnamon, stirring constantly, then the apples and pears. Arrange the sweet cream in the dessert bowls and sprinkle the chopped walnuts on each one.

BULGARIAN OAT CAKE

ingredients

for 4 people

50 g of butter 4 eggs a pinch of salt flour 150 g of sugar 150 g of oats 250 g of milk Beat the eggs with the sugar and a pinch of salt with a whisk or an electric mixer. Add the oatmeal by wetting it with a colander and stirring with a wooden spoon in an up and down motion. Add the melted butter, mix and put the mixture in a previously greased and floured mold; Bake in the oven for 35 minutes at a temperature of 180 °.

MALTAGLIATI DI OATS WITH FRESH GRASS, BACON AND PEAS

ingredients

for 4 people

for the pasta: 400 g of oats 4 eggs for the sauce: 1/2 glass of tomato sauce 4 tablespoons of extra virgin olive oil 5-6 fresh chives 1 jar of fine peas salt 100 g of bacon a sprig of parsley 100 g of grated Parmesan cheese salt and pepper Mix the oats with the eggs until a firm and well-worked dough is obtained, which is left to rest for about half an hour, then spread on a cutting board on a thin sheet.

With a pastry cutter, form irregular and irregular triangles, precisely maltagliati. Once the dough has been rolled out and cut, let it dry for half an hour so that it holds up better. Thinly slice the chives, add a few pieces of the stem and brown it in a pan with oil and diced bacon. Keep the heat very low. Add the peas and, after a few minutes, the tomato. Season with salt and pepper and cook over high heat for at least fifteen minutes, stirring. Cook the maltagliati separately, carefully, mix them with the sauce, mix them with the Parmesan cheese and decorate with the chopped parsley.

CAVATELLI WITH MUSHROOMS

INGREDIENTS:

500 g of mushrooms 400 g of cavatelli Parsley Garlic or shallot Cut the mushrooms into small pieces. In a pan, add 2 tablespoons of olive oil and a clove of garlic and the chopped shallot. Remove the garlic when it is golden. Add the mushrooms to the pan and brown them. Season with salt and pepper. Boil the cavatelli and, when they rise to the surface, pour them into the pan with the mushrooms. Mix the pasta well with the mushrooms and finally add the parsley.

SOUP CREAM,,
POTATOES WITH VEGETABLES

INGREDIENTS: 120 g of carrots 250 g of potatoes 80 g of pumpkin 120 g of cabbage 80 g of leek Chives Black pepper Thyme 1 clove of onion Celery Peel the carrots and potatoes and cut them into pieces. Clean the celery stalk and chop it. Chop the onion. Clean the leek and chop it. Wash the cabbage and chop the apple. Remove the seeds from the pumpkin and cut it into small pieces. In a pan pour a little oil and brown the celery, carrots, leek, and onion. As soon as they are wilted, add all the potatoes, cabbage and chives in succession, leaving them to flavor for a few minutes. Bring to a boil and simmer for 50 minutes, or until soft. When cooked, just before turning off, add the parsley and basil.

CREAM HOLDER E CHESTNUTS

INGREDIENTS:

2 leeks 1 potato 200 g chestnuts Half an onion 1 liter of water Parsley Basil Start by cooking the chestnuts in a saucepan with cold water for 10 minutes. Then petals and set them aside for now. Take another pot and start frying the onion with the oil. Add some basil, chopped onion and parsley. When the oil begins to brown, add the chestnuts, lower the heat a little and after 6 minutes add the chopped leeks. After another 5 minutes, pour the water into the mixture. Cover the pot and cook for another 40 minutes over low heat. When cooked, blend the mixture..

CHILI KITCHENS
ANGRY WITH ARTICHOKES

INGREDIENTS:

350 g of fettuccine 300 g of tomato pulp 3 artichokes 1 clove of garlic Parsley 40 black olives 2 peppers Chop the peppers, garlic, and parsley, then take a pan, pour a little oil, and add these ingredients. After a minute, finely chop the artichokes and add them to the pan, bring the water for the pasta to a boil. 2 minutes later, add the tomato and olives and simmer for 15 minutes. Skip the pasta, adjusting the cooking time. Add and add the pasta to the mixture and finally add the parsley if desired.

FETTUCCINE AL TARTUFO

INGREDIENTS:

400 g of fettuccine 1 clove of garlic or onion 100 g of truffle 60 g of butter Take a pan and start browning the garlic or onion (both if you want) with oil. When the oil is golden, add the butter. When you have finished browning well, remove the garlic. Start boiling the water. Clean the truffle well and cut it into very small slices. With the fire off, add the truffles to the mixture and mix well. Meanwhile, add the pasta, drain it a little before it is cooked, and pour it into the mixture, mixing well. If you want you can season it with another truffle or pepper or another spice of your choice.

MEXICAN STYLE CAULIFLOWER RICE

Preparation: 10 minutes
Cooking time: 15 min
Total time: 25 minutes
For: 4 people
ingredients
1 cauliflower
1 Onion
1 clove of garlic
3 tablespoons of tomato paste
1 teaspoon of oregano
½ spoonful of paprika
1 pinch of red pepper
Salt
and extra virgin olive
oil. Tools Food
processor

Cooking.

Finely chop the onion and sauté it together
with the garlic clove in a large pan with a
drizzle of oil for 5-6 minutes, adding a pinch of
salt. In the meantime, wash the cauliflower
well, divide it into florets and chop it for a few
seconds in the food processor just enough to
reduce it into coarse crumbs.

sauté the cauliflower
Add the tomato paste, chili, paprika,, and
oregano to the golden onion and sauté for a
couple of minutes. Then add the cauliflower,
season with salt and sauté for 5-7 minutes
until the cauliflower has softened a little but
has not lost its consistency. Serve
immediately hot or warm.

CHINESE RICE JOCKS WITH VEGETABLES, SHIITAKE AND ALMONDS

Preparation: 40 minutes
Cooking time: 10 min
Total time: 50 minutes
For: 4 people
ingredients
150 g of brown rice flour
50 g of type 0 flour
110 g of water 2 carrots
2 courgettes 2 chives
1 yellow pepper
shiitake mushrooms
soy sauce with almond salt
extra virgin olive oil
Cooking!
Shiitake mushrooms
Soak the shiitake mushrooms for at least 30 minutes. Coarsely chop the almonds. Sift the flours into a large bowl and pour in the water.

Knead until the water is completely absorbed and stop only when you have obtained a smooth and lump-free dough. Leave the dough to rest at room temperature for about 30 minutes wrapped in cling film. Cook the rice dumplings. After the resting time, take the dough and shape with your hands one or more sausages slightly flattened on the surface. From here cut into slices a few millimeters thick and flour again. Bring the water to a boil and cook the gnocchi by immersing them completely and collecting them with a skimmer after a few minutes, the cooking time will depend on how thin they are and when you want them al dente. They can usually cook for up to 10 minutes. The vegetables and we are ready. Cut the vegetables crosswise and brown them, together with the mushrooms, with extra virgin olive oil in a wok or non-stick pan until tender. Now season with soy sauce, a pinch of salt, and chopped fat almonds. Add the rice dumplings to the vegetables, season, and serve.

HIGH BANANA IN PROTEIN smoothie

Preparation time: 5 minutes Cook time: 0

minutes Number of servings: 2 Nutritional values

 per serving: Calories –608 Fat - 20 g carbohydrates

- 75 g of protein - 32 g of sodium - 301 mg Ingredients:

• 2 cups vanilla yogurt • 2 medium bananas, cut into pieces

• 4 scoops of protein powder

• 2 cups of

2% milk • 4 tablespoons of wheat germ How to use: 1. Place 2 large glasses in the freezer for 10 minutes.

2. Blend the yogurt, bananas, protein powders, milk, and wheat germ in a blender until smooth. 3. Pour

2 large, cold glasses and serve.

INTEGRAL BRETZEL

Preparation time: 20 minutes + rising time

Cooking time: 15 minutes per batch Number of servings: 28 Nutritional values per serving: Calories - 182 Fats - 2 Carbohydrates - 31 g Proteins - 10 g Sodium - 108 mg Ingredients: • 2 sachets of active dry yeast • 1 teaspoon of Kosher salt • 6 cups of whole wheat flour • 2 cups of bread flour • 1 cup of wheat gluten

• 4 tablespoons of baking soda • 4 teaspoons of brown sugar • 3 cups of warm water • 2 tablespoons of olive oil 2 egg whites or ½ cup of egg substitute • 2 tablespoons of sesame or poppy seeds or flax seeds or sunflower • 1/4 cups baking soda and 8 - 10 cups pretzel Cooking Instructions: 1. Put the dough hook in the mixer bowl if you want to knead the dough in the food processor. You can also work the dough in a bowl with your hands. 2. It is not possible to mix everything in the food processor at the same time, so prepare the dough twice. Pour the warm water into a bowl. Add yeast, salt and sugar. Set aside for 5 minutes. 3. Combine all the flour and form a bowl. Four.

bowl of the food processor. Pour half of the water mixture into the food processor along with half of the oil. 5. Work until the dough is formed. 6. Repeat steps 4 - 5 and prepare the remaining half of the dough. 7.

Spray 2 large bowls with cooking spray. Put a ball of dough in each bowl. Keep the container covered with cling film. 8. Place the bowls in a warm place for a couple of hours or until the dough rises and reaches twice its original size. 9. Prepare 2 baking sheets lined with parchment paper. 10. Pierce the dough with your fist. Divide the dough into 28 equal parts. 11. Roll out the dough, one at a time, held between the palms of the hands to form a long thread. Form a pretzel. Prepare the remaining pretzels in the same way.

12. Pour 8-10 cups of water into a saucepan. Put the saucepan over high heat. Add the baking soda and bring to a boil. 13. Dip the pretzels in boiling water, one at a time, and remove them after 30 seconds. 14. To remove, use a slotted spoon and place it on a baking sheet lined with parchment paper. 15. Brush the egg white or egg substitute over the pretzels. Sprinkle the pretzels with the chosen seeds. 16. Bake the pretzels in a preheated 450 ° F oven until golden brown, about 10-15 minutes.

BREAKFAST WITH PUMPKIN BREAD

Preparation time: 15 minutes Time cooking time: 30 minutes Servings: 4 Ingredients: 1/2 cup chopped walnuts 1 teaspoon baking powder 1 tablespoon lemon juice 1 tablespoon flaxseed flour 1 1/2 cup almonds 1 grated courgette 1 teaspoon of xanthan gum 1 tablespoon of butter, 3 eggs, melted, 1 teaspoon of beaten salt Instructions: preheat the oven to 180 ° C. In the bowl, combine all the wet ingredients. Beat the mixture well. Then add the baking powder, flax flour, almond flour, zucchini, xanthan gum and salt. Stir the mixture. Add the chopped walnuts and mix well. You will get a liquid but thick mixture. Check that you have added all the ingredients. Transfer the dough to a non-stick pan and level the surface with the spatula. Place the bread in the oven and bake for 50 minutes. Check if the bread is cooked with the help of a toothpick - if it is clean - the bread is cooked. Remove the courgette bread from the oven and let it cool well, then remove the pan from the pan and let it cool completely. Slice Lo.

MEDITERRANEAN FRITTATA

Preparation time: 5 minutes Time cooking time: 10 minutes Servings: 4 Ingredients: 3 beaten eggs 1 tablespoon of ricotta 2 oz. chopped feta cheese 1 chopped tomato, 1 teaspoon of butter, 1/2 teaspoon of salt, 1 tablespoon of chopped shallot Procedure: Mix the ricotta and eggs. Add salt and shallots. Fry the butter and let it melt. Pour 1/2 part of the beaten egg mixture into the pan and cook for 5-6 minutes or until the omelet is cooked through. Then transfer the tortilla to the plate. Prepare the second omelet with the remaining egg mixture. Sprinkle each tortilla with feta cheese and tomatoes. Rolled up. Nutrition: calories 203 Fats 15.2 Fibers 0.5 Carbohydrates 3.5

CREAMY OAT FLOUR WITH BANANA

Preparation time: 5 minutes Cooking time cooking: 10 minutes Servings: 4 Ingredients: 1 cup of berries of your choice 2 cups of oatmeal, 1 cup and 1/3 of sliced almonds 3 cups and 1/4 of water 1 tbsp. Ground cinnamon 2 medium bananas Procedure: Mash the bananas well until the mixture is smooth. Drain the water in a saucepan and add the banana puree. Combine the oatmeal in the pan and heat until the water boils. Set the burner temperature to minimum and continue heating for about 7 minutes. Remove from the heat and garnish with ground cinnamon, berri and sliced almonds. Serve immediately and enjoy your meal! Nutrition:

Calories: 265 Total Fat: 3 g Total Carbohydrates: 47 g Fiber: 5 g

PAN OF SHRIMPS

Preparation time: 10 minutes Time cooking time: 25 minutes Servings: 4 Ingredients: peppers 1 red onion 1 kg of peeled prawns 1/2 teaspoon of ground coriander 1/2 teaspoon of white pepper 1/2 teaspoon of paprika 1 tablespoon of butter Procedure: Remove the seeds from the peppers and cut the vegetables into wedges. Then put them in the pan. Add the peeled shrimp, white pepper, paprika,and butter. Peel and chop the red onion. Also, add it to the pan. Preheat the oven to 365F. Cover the pan with aluminum foil and close the edges tightly. Transfer to a preheated oven and cook for 20 minutes. After the time has elapsed, discard the aluminum foil and cook the dish for another 5 minutes, preferably in ventilated mode. Nutrition: Calories 153 Fats 4 Fibers 1.3 Carbohydrates 7.3 Proteins 21.5

TOMORROW "GRILL"

Preparation time: 10 minutes Time cooking time: 10 minutes
Servings: 4 Ingredients: 1 1/2 cup almond milk 1 cup whipping cream 4 tablespoons chia seeds 3 oz.

Grated Parmesan 1/2 teaspoon of red pepper flakes 1/2 teaspoon of salt 1 tablespoon of butter Procedure: Pour the almond milk into the saucepan and bring to the boil. Meanwhile, grind the chia seeds with the help of the coffee grinder. Remove the almond milk from the heat and add the ground chia seeds. Add the whipped cream, the red pepper flakes, and the salt. Mix well and leave for 5 minutes. At this point, add the butter and grated Parmesan. Mix well and preheat over low heat until the cheese has melted. bowls.

Nutrition: 439 calories 42.2 fat
Fiber 4.4 Carbohydrates 9.6 Proteins 10.7

BREAKFAST WITH MEAT

Preparation time: 10 minutes Cooking time: 30 minutes Yield: 4 Ingredients: 1 cup minced meat 1 cup chopped cauliflower 1/2 cup coconut cream 1 diced onion 1 teaspoon butter 1/2 teaspoon salt 1/2 teaspoon paprika 1/2 teaspoon garam masala 1 tablespoon chopped fresh cilantro 1 oz. celery root, grated 1 ounce. Grated cheddar cheese Procedure: Mix the mixture of garam masala, celeriac, paprika, salt, and ground beef. Mix the chopped cauliflower and salt. Brush the pan with butter. Place the ground beef mixture in the pan. Then arrange the layer of cauliflower and chopped onion. Sprinkle with grated cheese and fresh coriander, add the coconut cream. Cover the surface of the saucepan with cling film and close the lids. Preheat the oven to 365F. Place the pan in the oven and cook for 30 minutes. After the time has elapsed, remove the saucepan from the oven, remove the aluminum foil and let it cool for 15 minutes. Cut it into portions and transfer it to serve the bowls. Nutrition: Calories 192 Fats 14.7 Fibers 2.1 Carbohydrates 6.5 Proteins 10

OAT FLOUR, APPLES, AND SPICES

Ready in about: 15 min | Servings: 1 | Per serving: Kcal 190, Sodium 1 mg, Protein 5 g, Carbohydrates 39 g, Fats 2.5 g

INGREDIENTS 1 sweet apple, Gala type, peeled, cored, and cut into ½ inch cubes
⅔ cup of water ⅓ cup traditional oatmeal (rolled) a pinch of ground cinnamon a pinch of freshly grated nutmeg A few grains of kosher salt ½ cup skim milk, for serving

INSTRUCTIONS In a small saucepan, combine the water, apple, oats, nutmeg, cinnamon,, and salt. Bring to a boil over medium heat, reduce heat to low, and cover. Cook over low heat until the oatmeal is tender, about 4 minutes. Microwave: In a 1 liter microwave safe container, combine apple, water, oatmeal, cinnamon, nutmeg, and salt. You should cover it and microwave it on full power until the oats are tender for about 4 minutes. Cover carefully, mix and leave to rest for 1 minute. Transfer the oatmeal to a bowl, pour in the milk, and serve.

OAT FLOUR BAKED WITH APPLE CINNAMON

Ready in about: 50 min | Servings: 8 | Per serving: Kcal 312, Sodium 4 mg, Protein 9 g, Carbohydrates 60 g, Fats 7.5 g

INGREDIENTS 2 cups of steel cut oats 8 cups of water 1 tsp. cinnamon ½ tsp. allspice ½ tsp. nutmeg ¼ cup brown sugar 1 tsp. vanilla extract 2 apples, diced 1 cup raisins ½ cup unsalted walnuts, toasted, chopped

INSTRUCTIONS Spray the stove with non-stick cooking spray. Put all the ingredients on the stove except the walnuts. Mix well to combine. Put the pot on low heat for 30 minutes. Serve garnished with chopped walnuts.

YOGURT BANANA ALMONDS

Ready in about: 5 min | Portions:
1 per serving:
Kcal 337, Sodium 65mg, Protein 25

g, Carbohydrates 48 g, Fat 12 g

INGREDIENTS 1 tbsp. Unsalted Crunchy Raw Almond Butter ¾ cup of low-fat Greek yogurt, cup of old-fashioned raw oatmeal ½ teaspoon of sliced banana. cinnamon powder INSTRUCTIONS FOR USE Use the microwave to soften the almond for 15 seconds. Transfer the yogurt to a medium bowl and add the almond butter, oatmeal, and banana. Sprinkle with cinnamon.

BAKED EGGS BASIL AND TOMATO

**Ready in about: 25 min | Servings: 2 |
Per portion:
Kcal 235, Sodium 126 mg, Protein 14 g,**

Carbohydrates 7 g, Fats 16 g

**INGREDIENTS ½ clove of garlic, chopped
½ cup canned tomatoes ¼ cup fresh basil
leaves, coarsely chopped ¼ tsp. chili
powder ½ tbsp. olive oil 2 whole eggs
Pepper to taste**

**Preheat the oven to 180 ° C. Take a pan and
grease it with olive oil. Add the garlic, basil,
tomatoes, tomatoes, chili, olive oil to a plate and
mix. Break the eggs on a plate, leaving a space in
the center. Sprinkle the whole dish with sunflower
seeds and pepper. Place in the oven and cook for
12 minutes until the eggs have solidified and the
tomatoes are frothy. Serve with the basil on top.
Have fun!**

BLUEBERRY AND MAPLE OATMEAL

Ready in about: 30 min | Servings: 1 | Per serving: Kcal 260, Sodium 160 mg, Protein 9 g, Carbohydrates 49, Fats 3 g

INGREDIENTS ½ cup of rolled oats ½ cup of water or skim milk ⅛ tsp. sea salt 1 tbsp. chia seeds (optional) 1-2 tsp. maple syrup 2 cups of fresh blueberries

INSTRUCTIONS In a bowl or jar, combine the oatmeal, water or milk, and salt. Cover and refrigerate overnight. Before serving, decorate with chia seeds, Maple syrup Y blueberries

AMATRICO BUCATINI

INGREDIENTS:

200 g of pancetta 100 g of pecorino 400 g of bucatini 300 g of tomato pulp Collect the tomatoes and cut them into wedges. In a pan, heat the oil and add the chopped bacon and the chili. Brown the bacon until golden brown, then sprinkle with a little white wine. Let it evaporate, then turn off the heat and set the bacon aside. In the same pan put the cherry tomatoes and cook for the cooking time of the pasta.

When the pasta is almost cooked, add the pancetta to the sauce. Drain the pasta and put it in the pan with the sauce. Then season with grated pecorino and pepper.

LENTIL CREAM

INGREDIENTS:

200 g of pre-cooked lentils Half onion 1 carrot
Celery 2 cloves of garlic Cherry tomatoes Cut
the celery, onion, garlic and carrot, put them in
a saucepan with 2 tablespoons of oil. Fry for 1
minute and then add the cherry tomatoes. After
another minute, add the previously cooked
lentils. Add the saltwater a little at a time. Then
lower the heat and cook until the lentils are
soft. If it gets too dry, add more water. Before
blending everything, remove the remains of
garlic.

POTATO CREAM WITH VEGETABLES

INGREDIENTS:

120 g carrots 250 g potatoes 80 g pumpkin 120 g cabbage 80 g leek Chives Black pepper Thyme 1 onion Celery wedge Peel the carrots and cut the potatoes into pieces. Clean the celery stalk and cut it. Chop the onion. Clean the leek and chop it. Wash the cabbage and chop it. Remove the seeds from the pumpkin and cut them into small pieces. In a pan, add a drizzle of oil and fry the celery, carrot, leek, and onion. As soon as they are wilted, add all the potatoes, cabbage, and chives in succession, leaving them to flavor for a few minutes. Bring to a boil and simmer for 50 minutes, or until everything is smooth. When it is cooked, just before turning it off, add a little parsley and basil.

LEEK AND CHESTNUT CREAM

INGREDIENTS:

2 leeks 1 potato 200 g chestnuts Half an onion 1 liter of water Parsley Basil Start by cooking the chestnuts in a saucepan with cold water for 10 minutes. Then petals and set them aside for now. Take another pot and start frying the onion with the oil. Add some chopped basil, onion and parsley. When the oil begins to brown, add the chestnuts. Lower the heat a little and after 6 minutes add the chopped leeks. After another 5 minutes, pour the water into the mixture. Cover the pot and cook for another 40 minutes over low heat. When cooked, blend the mixture.

FETTUCCINE ANNOYED

WITH ARTICHOKES

INGREDIENTS:

350 g of fettuccine 300 g of tomato pulp 3 artichokes 1 clove of garlic Parsley 40 black olives 2 chillies Chop the peppers, garlic, and parsley, then take a pan, pour a little oil, and add these ingredients. After a minute, finely chop the artichokes and add them to the pan. Start boiling the water for the pasta. After 2 minutes add the tomato and olives and cook everything over low heat for 15 minutes. Add the pasta, adjusting for cooking. Add and mix the pasta well with the mixture and finally add a little parsley on top if you want.

ARTICHOKES FETTUCCINE

AND BACON

INGREDIENTS:

350 g of fettuccine 3 artichokes 150 g of bacon 1 clove of onion 1 clove of garlic Parsley Cream or other cheese (optional) Cut the artichokes and pancetta well. Take a pan and start browning the oil with the onion and garlic. After 2 minutes, add the bacon. Eliminate the garlic. Meanwhile, boil the water for the pasta. Add the artichokes and lower the heat a little. Cook for 12 minutes. Don't let the bacon burn. When cooked, pour it into the final mixture and add the parsley and pepper. You can also add cream or a piece of cheese or butter to make cream. Your turn.

GREEN FETTUCCINE WITH CHICKEN AND CHILEAN SAUCE

INGREDIENTS:

400 g of green pasta with eggs 60 g of pine nuts 1 slice of chicken breast 2 red peppers 70 g of parmesan A few mint leaves Cook the peppers for 15 minutes and blend. We take a pan and add the freshly made pepper cream together with the oil and salt. Add a ladle of cooking water. Cook over low heat. Boil the water for the pasta. In another pan, brown the chicken slice with the oil, then cut it finely when cooked. Chop the pine nuts and add them to the pepper mixture. If the pepper mixture has become too dry, add the cooking water. When it is almost cooked, add the pasta to the mixture and brown it, add the minced chicken, parmesan, and mint, and brown for about 3 minutes. Then serve it on the table.

RAVIOLI WITH RADICCHIO AND RICOTTA

ingredients

for four people: 300 g of flour 1 onion 450 g of
Treviso chicory 2 tablespoons of balsamic
vinegar of Modena 3 eggs oil 350 g of ricotta salt
150 g of grated Parmesan Pepper Shell 350 g of
chicory cut into thin strips and brown for 3
minutes in a pan, then cool. Sift the flour on a
pastry board, put the chicory, 2 eggs, two
tablespoons of water in the center, and work the
ingredients until the mixture is smooth and
homogeneous. Let it rest. Put the ricotta in a
bowl and mix it with 1 egg, 100 g of Parmesan,
then season with salt and pepper. Roll out half of
the dough into thin sheets and spread the
prepared filling in piles at regular intervals on
the surface, then lay the other half on the dough:
Crush the piles of filling with your fingers and
cut the ravioli with the pastry cutter. Chop the
onion and sauté it in a pan with five tablespoons
of oil, add the remaining radicchio into strips,
season with salt and pepper, and cook for 3
minutes. Cook the ravioli in boiling water,
garnish with the chicory sauce, sprinkle with
vinegar and serve.

PUMPKIN STUFFED WITH BEEF

INGREDIENTS

for four people: 6 fairly large courgettes 4 tablespoons of breadcrumbs 200 g of ground beef 6 thin slices of emmental 1 egg oil 2 tablespoons of milk Peel the courgettes and blanch them for 5 minutes in boiling water, then let them cool and cut them in half . sense of length: gently empty the pulp. Chop the zucchini pulp and put it in a bowl, then add the meat, milk, egg, and breadcrumbs, mix and fill the zucchini with the mixture. Place a thin slice on each courgette, sprinkle with breadcrumbs, put everything in a pan,and drizzle with oil. Bake in a preheated oven at 180 degrees for about 20 minutes and serve.

RIGATONI WITH MEATBALLS

INGREDIENTS

for four people: 400 g of rigatoni breadcrumbs 600 g of tomato pulp 1 egg 200 g of peas 70 g of grated Parmesan cheese 250 g of minced beef pulp garlic 1 onion salt 2 carrots oil butter In a bowl mix the meat and breadcrumbs , parmesan and egg: add salt and mix the ingredients. Form the meatballs and brown them in three tablespoons of oil flavored with a clove of garlic. When they are golden, we put them aside, add two tablespoons of oil and one of butter to the cooking sauce, brown the chopped onion and add the tomato pulp, season with salt and pepper, leave on the fire for 10 minutes and then add the meatballs. Cook over low heat for 20 minutes. Boil the diced carrots and peas and, in the meantime, also boil the rigatoni.

BEAN SOUP TO THE HAT

INGREDIENTS

for four people: 300 g of potatoes 4 chives 350 g of beans in candied chili sauce 1 liter of vegetable broth 3 red peppers oil 3 yellow peppers salt Toast the peppers for a few minutes on the grill, then peel and remove the filaments and seeds: cut into small pieces. Slice the chives and brown them in a saucepan for 3 minutes with four tablespoons of oil, then add the sliced potatoes, yellow peppers, and broth and cook over medium heat for 20 minutes. Blend the resulting soup and season with salt. In another saucepan, heat the beans with the red peppers: put the soup in individual bowls, and in each one put a spoonful of beans and peppers.

PASTA AND BEANS

INGREDIENTS

for four people: 250 g of cannellini beans with celery 250 g of different types of chili pasta 100 g of grated Parmesan cheese 4 ripe red tomatoes oil garlic salt basil Clean the beans and put them in a saucepan with 3 liters of cold water, cover and bring to a boil, then add the celery, the minced garlic and the basil, and the stale tomatoes through a sieve. Continue cooking and after 2 hours add the chopped bacon, red pepper, and five tablespoons of oil. Cook for another hour. Add the pasta and cook until al dente, add salt and serve with grated Parmesan and raw oil.

CABBAGE ROLLS

INGREDIENTS

for four people: 1 1 kg of cabbage 50 g of grated Parmesan cheese 150 g of rice boiled in medium flour 250 g of diced cooked ham butter 200 g of boiled and minced meat salt 2 eggs pepper medium chopped leek Put the cabbage in the cold and salted water on the stove, and boil for 10 minutes, then drain and cool. Explore the cabbage petals one by one. In a bowl combine all the other ingredients except the flour and butter, mix and pour a little on each cabbage leaf and fold them over themselves to form rolls. Y flour, brown in butter, then serve.

EGG MUFFINS FOR BREAKFAST

ingredients

1 cup diced broccoli Salt and

pepper {to taste} 8 eggs

1 cup onion, chopped

1 cup diced mushrooms

Instructions 1.

 Meanwhile, heat the oven to 350 degrees F. 2.

 Then cut all the vegetables into cubes.

you can add more or less, but keep the

 total portion of vegetables

the same for the best results. 3. After that, in a

 large bowl, beat the eggs, salt,

 greens and pepper. Four. Then pour the mixture

in a buttered muffin mold, the mixture should be

homogeneous and stuffed 8 molds for muffins

5. Now bake for 18-20 minutes, or until the

toothpick inserted in the center is clean. 6.

 Finally, serve and enjoy your meal! Leftovers

can be stored in the refrigerator for the

whole   week.

EASY AND DELICIOUS
SAUSAGE FRITTATA

Ingredients:

1 medium sweet potato {peeled and grated}

10 eggs Pepper

to taste}

1 pound Italian sweet sausage I

 used our fresh pork in the freezer)

4 green onions {chopped}

3 tablespoons of coconut oil

Instructions: 1 First, in a large skillet,

heat the coconut oil over medium heat.

It is then crumbled into the sausage (remember to remove it from the gut if necessary) and browned. 3. Next, add the grated sweet potato and cook until the potatoes are tender. Four.

Next, add the chopped green onion and sauté with the sausage and sweet potatoes for another 2-3 minutes.

5. Also, spread the sausage mixture evenly over the bottom of the pan. 6. Now beat the eggs and pour them evenly over the meat, sweet potato and spring onion.

blend. 7.This is when you spray it all over the place.

with black pepper. 8. Then, cook for approx

3 minutes or until boiling and you can see that the edges of

the   tortilla   that's how it is   almost
             cooked.

GRILLED VEGETABLES WITH PEANUT SAUCE

Preparation time:
10 minutes Cooking time:
30 minutes Servings: 4

INGREDIENTS: • 360 g of cauliflower florets • 360 g of broccoli flowers • 360 g of red cabbage (cut into small pieces) • 1 pepper (without seeds and membranes, chopped) • 1/4 tsp. salt and black pepper (each) • 1.5 kg boiled tofu (cut to 1.5 cm) • 2 tablespoons of peanut butter (powder) • 3 tablespoons of water

INDICATIONS:

Preheat the oven to 200 degrees. 2. Spread all the vegetables evenly on a lightly greased baking sheet and season with salt and black pepper. Grill until caramelized, but hold 3. Take a skillet and brown the tofu in a single layer until both sides are golden brown. To make a peanut sauce, take a bowl and whisk the powdered peanut butter and water together.

5. To serve, place the tofu in a bowl, garnish with the roasted vegetables and sprinkle with the peanut sauce Nutritional value: Energy (calories): 623 kcal - Protein: 64.98 g - Fat: 36.3 g - Carbon carbohydrates : 24.08 g

CAULIFLOWER SAUCE
CREAMY WITH SAUCE

Preparation time: 10 minutes
Cooking time: 20 minutes Servings: 4
INGREDIENTS: • 1 kg of
cauliflower florets • 60 g of cream
cheese (lean, softened) • 1 tbsp.
butter (unsalted, melted)
• 1 clove of garlic • 1 tablespoon of rosemary
• 1/4 teaspoon of salt • 1/4 tsp. Black
pepper • 3 tbsp. the mixture of sauces or
mushroom sauce • 180 g of cold water
HOW TO USE: 1. Put the water in a
saucepan and bring to the boil. Then boil
the cauliflower until it pierces easily with a
fork (about 10 minutes). Drain and let them
cool down a bit. 2. Add the cauliflower and
other ingredients to a blender and blend
until smooth. Prepare the sauce according
to the instructions on the package.
Nutrition: Energy value (calories):
90 kcal - Protein: 3.75 g - Fat: 5.76
g - Carbohydrates: 7.51 g

WHITE PIZZA WITH BROCCOLI CAKE

Preparation time: 10 minutes Cook time: 35 minutes Servings: 2

INGREDIENTS: • 750 g of broccoli • 1 egg of about 260 grated mozzarella (lean) • 60 g of grated Parmesan cheese • 1/2 tsp Italian seasoning • 120 g ricotta (partially skimmed) • 1/4 tsp. chili pepper • 1 clove of garlic (minced) • 120 g broccoli florets (chopped)

INSTRUCTIONS: 1. Preheat the oven to 200 ° C.. 2. Cook the broccoli in a microwave-safe saucepan and cover (about 3 minutes). 3. Once cool, transfer the broccoli to a clean, fine cloth or cheesecloth and squeeze to remove as much liquid as possible.

4. Take a bowl and combine the broccoli, egg, a third cup of mozzarella, Parmesan, and Italian dressing, then combine well.

5. transform the mixture into a square pizza (about 1 cm thick) on a baking sheet. Cook until the edges are golden brown (15-20 minutes).

6. Meanwhile, take a bowl and combine the ricotta, chili flakes, and garlic, then sprinkle this ricotta mixture over the broccoli crust, sprinkle with the remaining mozzarella, and add the broccoli. Cook again until the cheese has melted (about 5-10 minutes). Nutrition: Calories: 279 kcal - Protein: 23.85 g - Fat: 16.72 g-

Carbohydrates: 9.51 g

GREEN BEANS WITH GARLIC

Preparation time: 5 minutes Cook time: 10 minutes Servings: 4 ingredients • Green beans (with cut ends) - 680 g • Garlic and shallot dressing (or use a mixture of pepper, freshly chopped garlic, and salt) - 1 / 2 tablespoons • Toasted garlic oil (or other oil to taste) - 1 tablespoon • Parmesan (freshly grated) - 4 tablespoons Procedure: 1. Add the green beans to the saucepan. 2. Add about 2.5 cl of water to the pot. 3. Sprinkle with the dressing. 4. Cover the pot and put it on the stove. 5. Cook over high heat and simmer, about 7 minutes, or until the beans are fluffy, tender, and crunchy. 6. Drain the water and season with garlic, oil, pepper, and salt. 7. Sprinkle with Parmesan. To serve. Nutrition: Calories: 84 - Fat: 5g - Carbohydrates: 7.8g - Fiber: 3.7g - Sugar: 1.5g - Protein: 4g

ZOODLE DRESSED WITH GARLIC

Preparation time: 5 minutes Cooking time:

5 minutes Servings: 4

Ingredients: • Toasted garlic oil (or other oil to taste) - 1 tablespoon • Zucchini noodles - about 1 kg • Garlic and shallot dressing (or use a mixture of chopped fresh garlic, pepper and salt) - 1/2 tablespoon - With a pinch of salt and pepper Procedure: 1. With the pan, heat the oil over medium-high heat.
2. Add the courgette noodles and sprinkle with the dressing. 3. Cook for about 3 minutes. Jump from time to time. Season with a pinch of pepper and salt. To serve. Nutrition: Calories: 57 - Fat: 3.7 g
- Carbohydrates: 5.7 g - Fiber: 1.9 g - Sugar: 2.9 g - Protein: 2.1 g

SALMON FROM THE MEDITERRANEAN

Preparation time: 2 minutes
Cooking time: 12 minutes Servings: 4

ingredients • Wild salmon - 600g •
Mediterranean dressing - 1 tablespoon
Procedure: 1. Grease the pan with non-
stick cooking spray and heat over medium-
high heat. 2. Meanwhile, season the
salmon.
3. With the cut side facing down,
Put the salmon in the pan and brown it for
about 2 minutes. 4. Invert and turn the
heat down to medium. 5. Cover the pan
and cook for another 6 minutes or until the
salmon is completely cooked. 6. Then
serve. Nutrition: Calories: 188 - Fat: 8.8 g -
Carbohydrates: 0 g - Fiber: 0 g - Sugar: 0 g
- Protein: 27.5 g

PASTA WITH PESTO CHICKEN WITHOUT FAT AND VEGETABLES

Preparation time: 5 minutes
Cooking time: 15 minutes Servings: 1

INGREDIENTS: • 3 cups of raw cabbage leaves • 2 tablespoons of olive oil • 2 cups of fresh basil • 1/4 teaspoon of salt
• 3 tablespoons of lemon juice •3 cloves of garlic • 2 cups of cooked chicken breast
• 1 plate of spinach • 170 g of raw chicken noodles
• 85 cubes of fresh mozzarella • basil leaves or chili flakes for garnish

INDICATIONS:

Start by making the pesto, add the cabbage, lemon juice, basil, garlic cloves, olive oil, and salt in a blender and blend until smooth. 2. Add pepper to taste. 3. Cook the pasta and drain the water. Reserve 1/4 cup of liquid. 4. Take a bowl and mix everything together, the cooked pasta, the pesto, the minced chicken, the spinach, the mozzarella, and the reserve liquid of the pasta. 5. Sprinkle with more chopped basil or chili flakes (optional). 6. Your salad is ready. You can serve it hot or cold. In addition, it can be eaten as a mixed salad or as a garnish. Leftovers should be stored in the refrigerator in an airtight container for 3-5 days. NUTRITION: Calories: 244 - Protein: 20.5 g - Carbohydrates: 22,

LIGHT SMOKE
WITH VEGETABLES

Preparation time: 5 minutes Cook time: 0 minutes Servings: 1

INGREDIENTS: • 1/2 cup of cabbage leaves • 3/4 cup of cold apple juice • 1 cup chopped pineapple • 1/2 cup frozen green grapes • 1/2 cup sliced apple INSTRUCTIONS: 1. Put the pineapple, apple, juice, apple, frozen seedless grape, and cabbage leaves in a blender. 2. Close and mix until smooth. 3. The smoothie is ready and can be garnished with halved eggs if desired.

NUTRITION: Calories: 81 - Proteins: 2 g - Carbohydrates: 19 g - Fat: 1 g

PU SOUP, PUMPKIN, AND

PUMPKIN Ingredients:

250 grams pumpkin 250gr. onions 4-5 large mushrooms 2 cloves of garlic 3-4 tbsp. sour cream 1 shallot onion 100 ml. dry white wine 800 ml. Pottage
1 tablespoon butter salt herbs lemon juice - to taste

Preparatio

Clean the pumpkin and courgettes and cut them into cubes. Chop the shallot and garlic and fry with half the butter until transparent, add the pumpkin, courgettes, and cook, stirring, for 5 minutes. Deglaze with the wine and cook for 1-2 minutes over high heat. Add the broth and simmer, over low heat, for 20 minutes under the lid. Then mix the soup with a blender, add lemon juice to taste, salt and pepper, add sour cream and heat, do not boil. Superior. Chop the mushrooms and fry them in the remaining oil for 2-3 minutes, add the aromatic herbs, salt, and pepper. Serve the soup, put the mushrooms in the center with the aromatic herbs.

PUMPKIN SOUP WITH

CHICKEN Ingredients:

400 grams a pumpkin 1 small leek 2 carrots 2 onions 8 slices of bacon 8 potatoes 3-4 tbsp. vegetable oil salt pepper provencal herbs bay leaf cumin sesame - to taste

Preparation:

Wash the chicken, peel it, cover it with cold water, add salt, add the bay leaf, carrot, pepper and cook the soup. Cut the pumpkin and potatoes into cubes, add the aromatic herbs, cumin,l,and chili pepper to taste and cook in a little salted water. Fry the bacon in a non-stick pan, remove and brown the onions in the remaining fat until golden brown. Using a chicken carcass, remove the meat and slice it. The vegetables are boiled with the help of a mixer. Add the meat, heat a little and pour into the dishes. On each plate put the slices of bacon, the fried onion and sprinkle with sesame seeds.

SALMON IN LEMON JUICE

Ingredients:

1 kilogram. salmon 3-4 lemon 2-3 tbsp. vegetable oil 1 pc. sugar black pepper salt and fresh ginger - to taste

Preparation:

Squeeze the juice from the lemons, crumble them with the help of a small grater, add salt, pepper, grated ginger, sugar, and a little cold boiled water. Salmon on skewers and marinate in the resulting mixture in 2 h. This barbecue is best fried on the grill. Preheat the barbecue marinade and water while cooking.

SALMON AND SPINACH PACKAGING

Ingredients:

Salmon fillets (1 per serving)
Fresh Spinach Fresh Lemon

Preparation:

Wash and dry the salmon portions ... Sprinkle each portion with a small piece of butter. Carefully wrap in fresh spinach leaves. Tie the packages together with string. Cook the meatballs for 20 minutes.

6. Serve with lemon wedges.

PUMPKIN SOUP WITH SMOKED FISH

Ingredients:

500 grams of smoked fish 500 gr. a pumpkin 3 potatoes 2 tomatoes 1 onion 1 carrot 200 ml. 10-20% cream 1 teaspoon. Paprika mix Salt - al taste

Preparation:

Purified pumpkin, potatoes, carrots and onions cut into cubes and boiled in salted water for 5-7 minutes. Put it in a colander. Cut the tomatoes crosswise, drain them with boiling water, cool them immediately in ice water, and remove the skin. Pass the cooked vegetables and tomatoes through a colander and pour them into the pan. Divide the fish along the ridge, remove all the bones. 1 rib of sirloin, the second cut pcs. Add the fish to the vegetables in a pan, pour the cream, stir, bring to a boil and immediately remove from the heat. Add the spices, cover,was and leave rest for 10 minutes.

PUMPKIN SOUP WITH SPICES AND ORIENTALS

Ingredients:

1 small pumpkin 2 onions 1 clove of garlic 1.5 liters of vegetable broth 1 bay leaf 1 tsp. brown sugar 1-2 tsp. curry powder 0.5 tsp. ground cinnamon 0.25 tsp. ground nutmeg 1 tsp.

Plain yogurt or low-fat sour cream

Salt ground black pepper with

herbs - to taste.

Preparation:

The pumpkin cut in half and placed on a baking sheet. Onions are cleaned from the skin and cut into quarters. Unpeeled garlic, wrapped in aluminum foil. Place the vegetables in the pan and bake at 180 ° C for 1 hour. Allow to cool slightly, scrape the pumpkin pulp into a pot, squeeze the garlic from the peel and add the onion and whisk until smooth. Add the broth, spices to taste, bring to a boil and simmer for 10 minutes. Get out of the fire; add sour cream e

FAST FISH CAKE

Ingredients:

400 grams of fish filets 1-2 onions 1 tsp. mayonnaise 1 tsp. our cream 2 eggs 0.5 tsp. soda 0.25 tsp. vinegar 1 tsp Flour Salt Spices for fish dishes Preparation: Mix sour cream, mayonnaise and vinegar. Flour connects with soda.

Setting up

a mixture of sour cream, flour, and egg batter. The fish filets are cut into portions. Pour half of the batter into the prepared pan, lay a fish, lay the onion rings or half rings on top, and pour the remaining batter. Bake at 200 ° C until golden brown.

RABARBER CRUMBLE RECIPE

The rhubarb crumble is a real one popular Find out how to do the

rhubarb crumbling after this simple recipe.

Ingredients:

12 stalks of rhubarb 4 tbsp. Water 8 tbsp. Sugar 110 gr. Butter (minced) 110 gr. Sugar 180 gr. Preparation of the flour:

Preheat the oven to 180 ° C. Cut the rhubarb into 5 cm-2 inch pieces. Put the rhubarb, water and sugar in a saucepan. Put the butter, flour, and sugar in a bowl and mix well until you get a soft sand. Place the flour mixture on top of the rhubarb and cook for 45 minutes - 1 hour until golden brown. Serve hot with ice cream.

RICE CAKE WITH PLUMS.

Ingredients:

Soft wheat flour 60gr. • Rye flour 150 gr. • Cane sugar 150 gr. • Butter 150 gr. • New 3 pieces. • 1 teaspoon of baking powder. • Plum 10 units. • 1 tablespoon of powdered sugar. Preparation:

Step 1: Soften the oil with sugar.

Step 2 Add one egg at a time, after each.

Step 3 Let's add two types of sifted flour and yeast.

Step 4. We mix everything well, the dough turns out like thick sour cream.

Step 5 Cover the 19-20 cm mold with baking paper, pour the mixture, and place half of the chopped and dried plums on top.

Step 6 Bake at 190 * until cooked, about 45-50 mins.

Step 7: Sprinkle the cake with powdered sugar. Step 8: drink good tea.

RECIPE OF ROASTED BEET

Roasted beetroot is a very popular recipe. Find out how to make roasted beets by following this simple recipe.

Ingredients:

8 fresh beets 3 tbsp. Extra virgin olive oil 1 tablespoon. Sea salt 2 jets. thyme

Preparation:

Preheat the oven to 400 ° F. Wash the beets in cold water and dry them. Remove the shard, leaving at least 1 stalk or a little more. Put the beets in a pan, boil the beets well. Sprinkle the greased beets with salt and thyme. Roast the beets in a preheated oven for about 40-45 minutes or until soft. Cool the beets and gently peel them with tissue paper. Remove the stems. Serve hot with goat cheese or other

"REAL" SALAD WITH PLUMS

Ingredients:

2 chicken breasts 6 cooked potatoes 5
hard-boiled eggs 1 bunch of shallots
300 gr. dried plums 300 gr. aged cheese
1 tomato with olive mayonnaise
herbs

Preparation:

Peel the eggs and potatoes, boil the chicken,
separate the yolks from the whites, the onion
and chop the plums with a knife. Chicken:
disassemble the fibers, rub the potatoes on a
coarse grater, cheese - on a fine. Arrange on a
plate: chicken, mayonnaise, onions, potatoes,
mayonnaise, onions, plums, mayonnaise,
cheese, grated egg yolk, mayonnaise, roll, and
grated protein. Garnish with slices of tomato
salad, olives, herbs and leave to soak for 30
minutes.

SALAD OF BROCCOLI AND APPLES

Ingredients:

300 grams broccoli 100 gr. apple 1 lemon

50 grams. dill olive oil salt

Preparation:

Rinse the broccoli under running cold water, separate the inflorescences and soak them in boiling salted water for 3 minutes. Finely chopped dill apples cleaned and thinly sliced. Lemon Wash and cut with the peel into very thin slices. Mix all the ingredients and dress the salad with olive oil. Breakfast: The most important meal of the day, but some people prefer not to have breakfast due to lack of time. We offer 2 light but hearty broccoli dishes that can be served for breakfast and for cooking, which doesn't take long: broccoli in a cheese omelet, and broccoli in a green garlic tempura.

BRUSSELS SPROUTS SALAD WITH TOMATO AND CHILE

Ingredients:

400 grams Brussels sprouts 100 gr. Tomatoes 100 grams pepper 100 gr. green onions 1 onion 3 tablespoons vegetable oil 1

lemon sugar ground black

pepper - to taste Preparation:

Each head cut into slices, onion cut into half rings, green onions - strips. Sliced tomatoes and peppers. Combine all the vegetables, pour in the lemon juice and refrigerate for 2 hours. Then season the salad with sugar, ground black pepper to taste, season with vegetable oil and mix.

CABBAGE SALAD WITH CARROTS AND BEETS

Ingredients:

200 grams of cabbage 1 beetroot 1 carrot 1 bunch of green onions 1 Teaspoon. 1 tbsp wine vinegar. sesame oil 1 tsp. mustard salt in grains - to taste **Preparation:**

Carrots and beets are cut into thin strips or rubbed on a fat Korean salad, the cabbage is chopped, lightly sautéed, and resembles hands. Green onions are cut into rings. Mix all the ingredients, dress the salad with the mixture of sesame oil, vinegar, mustard and salt.

CHILDREN WITH ALGAE

ingredients

300 g of flour 0
300 g of warm water
chopped spoons
dry seaweed
1 teaspoon of salt
3 g of brewer's yeast
dry frying oil
Cooking!
Pour the flour into a bowl and mix
salt and seaweed, then add the brewer's yeast
and start pouring the lukewarm water,
kneading everything with your hands until
you get a smooth dough. Knead for a few
minutes with your hands, then cover with
cling film and
let it rise for about 3 hours in a
warm place away from the
temperature. To fry

When the dough has doubled in volume, put a high pan on the stove and fill it with oil for frying. When the oil is hot, take some of the dough with a spoon and gently slide it into the oil, helping yourself with a second spoon. Cook the pancakes for a few minutes, until they are golden brown and well cooked inside (you can first test to see that the oil temperature is good), then gradually drain them with a slotted spoon and place them on a plate. Absorbent paper to remove excess oil. Continue cooking your zeppole until the pasta is cooked and served immediately, hot, so you can enjoy the fragrant and crunchy.

POTATO CAKE

Preparation: 20 minutes
Cooking: 90 minutes
Total time: 1 hour and 50 min
For: 4 people

ingredients

1 kg of potatoes
50 g of baby spinach
5 g of nutritional yeast
10 g of salt
1 teaspoon of pepper
thyme breadcrumbs to taste
Tools: potato masher, blender, baking
pan Cooking! water and serve the
abundant salty water
to consume Skins approx.

As soon as they are tender, listen to them and let them cool. Meanwhile, put the spinach, nutritional yeast, and spices in a blender and blend until smooth. Using a potato masher, mash the potatoes until they are pureed. Now add everything and mix to mix the ingredients well, then season with salt. In the oven, grease a ceramic pan and sprinkle the surface and edges with breadcrumbs. Pour the mashed potatoes and level with a ladle, sprinkle with a generous handful of breadcrumbs and bake at 180 degrees for about 40 minutes, taking care to grill for the last 5 minutes.

MINI QUICHE OF PUMPKIN WITH MINT AND PISTACHIOS

Preparation: 15 minutes
Cooking: 40 minutes
Total time: 55 minutes
For: 4 people
ingredients
1 roll of wholemeal puff pastry
120 g of unsweetened soy milk
2 courgettes
60 g of pistachios
15 g of chickpea flour (1 tablespoon)
1 teaspoon of mustard
1 teaspoon of nutritional yeast
1 sprig of mint
1 clove of garlic
food processor tools 4 cupcake cases with a diameter of 10 cm Cooking time! fry the zucchini
Wash and cut the courgettes into fairly thin slices. In a pan, sauté lightly

the garlic clove with a little extra virgin olive oil until golden brown. Pour in the courgettes and cook over high heat for 5 minutes, until they begin to soften. Turn off the heat and season with salt, pepper and mint cut into strips. We prepare the cream. Pour the tofu, unsweetened soy milk, chickpea flour, mustard and nutritional yeast into a food processor and blend until smooth and homogeneous. Transfer the cream to a bowl and add the coarsely chopped courgettes and pistachios. Mini filling for quiche Line the molds with the puff pastry, prick the bottom with the tip of a fork and fill each one with the filling. Bake in a static oven at 180 ° C for 35-40 minutes on the lower grill of the oven,

THOUSAND-SHEET POTATO CAKE

INGREDIENTS
800 g of raw potatoes already cleaned
150 g of breadcrumbs
2 tablespoons of pecorino or other
cheese to taste
dry rosemary to taste
optional chili powder
salt and oil to taste
300 g of sliced provolone
PROCESSES
Clean the potatoes and cut them into very
thin slices with a mandolin. Put them in a
container full of cold water and leave
them to infuse for about 10 minutes. In
this way they will lose some of their
starch, it will not darken and after
cooking they will be nice and crunchy.
In a bowl, prepare the breadcrumbs and
mix it with the dried rosemary and
pecorino.

I recommend adding some chili powder, but this step is optional. Prepare a 24 cm diameter cake pan and grease the bottom and edges with olive oil. Spread the breadcrumb mixture on the bottom. Drain the potato slices and start distributing them one by one on the bottom to form the first layer. Add the salt and a layer of breadcrumbs, the olive oil and a few slices of provolone. We form a second layer of potatoes and proceed in this way until all the ingredients are used up. Bake at 180 degrees for about 50 minutes. Eventually the potatoes will be crunchy on the surface. Let it cool for a few minutes and open the pan. Chop the potato mille feuille and serve it hot. Try it yourself!

POTATO CRUMBOLA

Preparation time: 30 minutes
Cooking time: 35 minutes
Ready in: 1 hour and 5 minutes
INGREDIENTS
FOR THE MASS
600 g of potatoes
1 egg 180 g of flour 00
40 g of grated cheese
Salt to taste
2 tablespoons of breadcrumbs
Pepper as needed
FOR THE STUFFING
2 sausages
200 g of sliced mozzarella for pizza
PROCESSES
First boil the potatoes in boiling water
and, in the meantime, fry half an onion
cut into strips in a pan with olive oil. Add
the chopped sausage. Check with a fork
that the potatoes are soft and drain them.
To crumble them we have two options:
we can peel and mash them with a fork or
use a potato masher.

Add salt, one egg and mix well.
While continuing to mix, add the
grated cheese and flour. Our
crumbled dough is ready!
We take an opening mold and cover the
bottom with baking paper. Cover the base
with the potato mixture, pressing with your
hands to compact it. Pour the onion and
sausage filling into the base and add the
diced mozzarella for pizza. Cover
everything with the excess dough, taking
small pieces with your hands and spreading
it on the surface. In this way we will create
potato curls that will remain crunchy during
cooking. Complete with a pinch of
breadcrumbs and a little pepper. Bake the
potato crumble in the oven for 35 minutes at
200 °. Our potato crumb is ready, the filling
is delicious and the surface is golden and
crunchy!

TUNA AND POTATO FLAN

Preparation time: 5 min
Cooking time: 40 minutes
 Ready in: 45 min
DOSE FOR 8 PORTIONS
INGREDIENTS
1 kg of boiled potatoes
300 g of tuna in oil
(weight once drained)
50 g of grated cheese
(like parmesan or parmesan) 2
eggs Salt and pepper to taste
Parsley Breadcrumbs to taste
Olive oil to taste
METHOD
In a large bowl, mash the potatoes with the
help of a potato masher, then add the eggs,
well-drained tuna, grated cheese, a sprig of
chopped parsley, pepper, and a pinch of
salt.

In a large bowl, mash the potatoes with a
potato masher, add the eggs, the drained
tuna, the grated cheese, a sprig of chopped
parsley, the pe,pper, and a pinch.

of salt. In a large bowl, mash the potatoes with a potato masher, then add the eggs, drained tuna, grated cheese, a sprig of chopped parsley, pepper, and a pinch of salt. Mix all ingredients until well blended. Mix all ingredients until well blended. Transfer the freshly made mixture to a pan greased with breadcrumbs (mine measures 22cm x 22cm). Level the mixture with slightly moistened hands, then decorate the surface by rubbing with the tines of a fork. Sprinkle with little breadcrumbs, sprinkle with a drizzle of oil and bake in a preheated oven at 180 ° for 40 minutes, perhaps activating the "grill" function for 5 minutes before removing the flan from the oven.

FRENCH FRIES TOAST

Preparation time 15 min
 Cooking time: 30 min
 Ready in: 45 min
DOSAGE FOR 4/5 TOAST
INGREDIENTS
3-4 medium boiled potatoes
3-4 tablespoons of breadcrumbs
a tablespoon of olive oil a sliced
cheese egg Salt to taste; onion
to taste
PROCESSES
First we start by boiling the potatoes and
then let them cool completely. Remove
the skin and mash them well with a fork.
We add an egg and continue to mix the
mixture well, adding the chives, salt, and
a little oil. You can use your favorite
spices to enrich the mixture such as
paprika, rosemary, turmeric, etc.

We also add 3-4 tablespoons of breadcrumbs, take a sheet of baking paper and sprinkle with a little breadcrumbs. We take some dough and start forming our toast. Let's try to give it a square shape. Once the base of the toast was obtained, stuffed with cheese to taste, I used a little sliced cheese but it is excellent to use slices of mozzarella. Close the toast with another square of potatoes and add some breadcrumbs on top. Once the base of the toast has been prepared, fill it with cheese to taste. I used some sliced cheese but it's fine if you want to stuff it with slices of mozzarella. We close the toast with another square of potatoes and add little breadcrumbs to the surface. Heat a grill with a little oil and cook the toasts for 5-6 minutes per side,

POTATO CROQUETTES
WITH A FUN HEART

INGREDIENTS

500 g of boiled potatoes
1 egg
60 g of grated Parmesan cheese
50 g of breadcrumbs
12-15 mozzarella
salted oil for frying
FOR THE CRUMBS
00 flour to taste 1 egg
breadcrumbs to taste
PROCESSES
Boil the potatoes in boiling water, peel, and mash them. Let them cool and add the beaten egg, Parmesan, breadcrumbs, and salt.

Mix to obtain a homogeneous mixture. Now let's go and shape the croquettes: take a little dough, flattened in the palm of your hand, and put a little mozzarella inside. Close the dough and form a ball. Once all the croquettes have been prepared, pass them first in the flour, then in the beaten egg, and finally in the breadcrumbs. In a pan we heat the oil for frying, to see if it is ready just wet a wooden stick and if it boils, we can start. Fry a little at a time, turning the croquettes on all sides. When they are golden, we drain them on absorbent paper, then we arrange them in a sauce and we are ready to serve!

SHORT SLEEVES
TUNA AND OLIVES

DOSE FOR 4 PEOPLE

ingredients

150 grams of tuna
100 grams of green olives.
Half sleeves of 350 grams. 1/2
red onion
to the taste of olive oil
processes
Boil 350 g of half sleeves in salted water. In
a large pan, fry half a thinly sliced red onion
in olive oil. Add the tuna and sauté for a few
minutes, then add the green olives cut in
half. Drain the pasta and add it to the sauce
in the pan, stir in for a few seconds, and
ready to serve!

CHICKEN WITH PEPPERS

Cooking time: 50 min
 Ready in: 50 min
dose for 4 people

INGREDIENTS

3 cloves of garlic
3 tablespoons of extra virgin olive oil 1
chicken cut into pieces (1 kg / 1.5 kg)
1/2 glass of white wine
1 glass of water
1 red pepper
1 yellow pepper
2 sprigs of rosemary
Salt to taste
PROCESSES
Pour the oil into a pan and add the minced chicken. Add two or three cloves of garlic (I don't hear them) and cook for 5 minutes, stirring occasionally.

Add the wine and half a glass of water and cook with the lid on for about 40 minutes, remembering to stir from time to time. During cooking, if necessary, add another half glass of water. In the meantime, wash and cut the peppers in half to remove the seeds, then cut them into strips. When the liquid has been absorbed, add the peppers cut into strips, add the sprig of rosemary, and season. Cook for another 5 minutes, stirring occasionally. Chicken with peppers should be served hot, sometimes I bring it to the table right in the pan!

BAKED STUFFED CHICKEN BREAST ROLL

Preparation time 10 min
Cooking time: 40 minutes
 Ready in: 50 min
It serves 6
ingredients
PROCESSES
Spread a sheet of parchment paper on the work surface and place the slices of chicken breast on top, overlapping them slightly, to form a fairly regular rectangle. Season with salt and pepper to taste. Start filling the chicken roll with the slices of cooked ham until it covers the entire surface, leaving the flap that will correspond to the closure free. It is important to start stuffing with the ham as it will give "structure" to the roll and will form a sort of inner sleeve for all the other ingredients.

Continue to stuff with the slices of mozzarella. Continue to stuff with the sautéed and well-squeezed spinach, then finish by arranging the hard-boiled eggs. Now roll up the chicken slices on themselves embracing the filling, helping with the baking paper to form a very compact loaf and compact roll. Tie the roll with some rosemary and sage leaves with kitchen twine, making the knots firmly. Season the roll with another pinch of salt and pepper, sprinkle with wine and finally sprinkle with olive oil. Bake the roll in a convection oven at 180 ° for 35-40 minutes, brushing it from time to time with your cooking juices. When the roll is cooked, let it cool for about ten minutes, then remove the kitchen string and cut it into slices, not too thin. serve the

STRIPS OF CHICKEN SAFFRON AND PUMPKIN

INGREDIENTS
1 medium courgette
500 g of chicken breast
1/2 onion in olive oil
Flour
1 saffron 1/2 glass of milk
PROCESSES
Wash and chop a medium-sized courgette.
Cut the chicken breast into strips and flour it
in a bowl. In a pan, chop half an onion and
add the olive oil. Brown the onion and add
the chopped courgettes. Let it cook for a few
minutes, stirring occasionally. Add the
marinated chicken strips and cook, stirring
often. Also, dissolve a bag of saffron in half a
glass of milk. Pour into a pan, season with
salt,,, and cook covered, stirring occasionally,
until the liquid is absorbed. The chicken
strips with courgettes and saffron are ready
to be served! Enjoy your meal!

BAKED FRITTATA WITH ,POTATOES AND ONIONS

Preparation time: 5 min
Cooking time: 35 min
Ready in: 40 min
NEEDS 6

INGREDIENTS

500 grams of potatoes 1 large onion
4 eggs 50 g of grated Parmesan
cheese Half a glass of milk
Salt and pepper to taste
Rosemary to taste Extra virgin
olive oil to taste

PROCESSES

In a saucepan put the potatoes cut into
medium thickness slices and the onion
cut into thick slices. Season with salt,
pepper, a few sprigs of rosemary, and a
drizzle of oil. Pour in a cup of water, put
the lid on and cook the potatoes for 15-20
minutes.

However, be careful not to let them overcook and fall apart. Peel the eggs in a large bowl and add the grated Parmesan and milk. Add a pinch of salt and mix everything with a whisk or fork until the mixture is smooth. Add the potatoes to the egg mixture and mix gently. Transfer the mixture to a baking tray lined with parchment paper and, if necessary, evenly distribute the potato slices. Place the pan in a preheated oven at 180° for 30 - 35 minutes, making sure that the tortilla is well cooked with the typical test of cotton candy. Here is the baked omelet with potatoes and onions served at the table! I recommend accompanying it with a rich mixed salad.

CASH CHEESE WITH BLUEBERRIES AND PUMPKIN SEEDS

Preparation: 10 min (+ 2 hours and 30 minutes of rest) Total time: 10 min (+ 2 hours and 30 minutes of rest) ingredients
150 g of raw cashews
1 ½ tablespoon of yeast
Nourishing juice of ½ lemon
1 teaspoon of mustard
1 pinch of salt
1 pinch of garlic powder
1 pinch of pepper
30 g of blueberries
20g Pumpkin Seed Food Processor Tools

Cooking.

Soak the cashews in warm water for 2 hours, then listen to them stunned in the food processor and add the nutritional yeast, lemon juice, mustard, salt, pepper and garlic powder. If you don't like cashews, you can try using almonds or macadamia nuts. Mix everything well until the mixture is smooth, transfer it to a bowl, and add 20 g of very coarsely chopped cranberries. We shape our cheese. Line a large, shallow bowl with cling film and pour the cashew mixture into it, pressing down well. Cover the edges with cling film and let it rest in the refrigerator for at least 30 minutes. Decorate the surface Once ready, remove it from the bowl and remove the film,

GRAPE TRUFFLE AND SALTED TOFU WITH PISTACHIOS AND WALNUTS

Preparation: 15 minutes
Total time: 15 minutes
For: 8 people
ingredients
300 g of tofu
300 g of black and white grapes
30 g of almond flour
30 g of walnut flour
50 g of chopped walnuts
50 g of chopped pistachios
3 tablespoons of extra virgin olive
oil Juice of ½ lemon Chili Utensils
Food processor Cook!

First, dry the tofu well with
absorbent paper to remove as
much water as possible,

then blend in the food processor together with the almond and walnut flour (you can easily prepare them at home by beating the same amount of walnuts in the food processor until you get the finest flour possible). Add the oil, lemon juice, salt and a pinch of red pepper and mix again until you get a smooth and fairly firm cream. Shape the truffle

Wash and dry the grapes well, then coat each grape with 1 tablespoon of tofu cream to form an even layer. Pass the black grape balls into the pistachio grains, and the white grape balls into the walnut grains. Place them on a tray or serving dish and let them rest in the refrigerator for at least an hour before serving.

CHICKPEAS FRUIT WITH HERBS AND CAULIFLOWER MAYONNAISE

Preparation: 10 min Cooking time: 15 min
Total time: 25 minutes
It serves approx. 18 pancakes
ingredients
120 g of flour 0 40 g of chickpea flour
125 g of cooked chickpeas
1 teaspoon of cream
natural tartaric yeast
1 teaspoon of rosemary, chopped
½ teaspoon of chopped sage
160 g unsweetened soy milk
Salt and pepper Oil for frying 1
dose of cauliflower
mayonnaise Cooking.

First, in a bowl, mix the 0 flour with the chickpea flour, baking powder, rosemary, sage, salt, and pepper and mix well with a whisk. At this point, add the soy milk a little at a time, mixing with a whisk until the dough is smooth and not too thick.

You fill the dough

Coarsely chop the chickpeas with a knife and add them to the mixture. In a high-sided saucepan, pour plenty of oil for frying and heat. Check that it has reached the right temperature by pouring a few drops of batter into the oil: they should rise to the surface in 2-3 seconds. Let's fry! Start frying by pouring a spoonful of batter at a time into the boiling oil without filling the pan too much to avoid lumps and pancakes, and cook until golden brown. Drain them with a slotted spoon and drain the excess oil on a plate covered with absorbent paper. Continue in this way to fry a few pancakes at a time until the mixture is used up. Serve immediately hot and crunchy, accompanied by cauliflower mayonnaise.

NOODLES WITH SOY SAUCE

Preparation: 15 minutes

Cooking: 60 minutes
Total time: 1 hour 15 min
For 6 people
ingredients
500 g of noodles without egg
80 g of soy granules
150 g of mixed vegetables for
sautéing (celery, carrot, onion)
400 g of tomato pulp
100 ml of red wine 1 clove of garlic
1 tablespoon of aromatic herbs of Provence
2 bay leaves
1 tablespoon of tomato paste
1 homemade vegetable cube
2 tablespoons of soy sauce (optional)
Vegetable broth Nutmeg Salt and
pepper Cook.
Take care of the soy grains first.
Bring about 1.5 liters of
vegetables to a boil.

Broth in a saucepan, lightly salt, and boil the soy granules for about ten minutes, then drain and set aside.

Let's prepare the ragù base, let's now move on to the vegetables for the sauté: wash and clean them well, then cut them into very small cubes. In a large pot, heat a drizzle of oil with the minced garlic clove, bay leaves, and Provencal herbs and leave to flavor for a couple of minutes. Add the drained soy granules, cook for a couple of minutes and then deglaze with the red wine. We complete the ragù

Add the vegetable cube, tomato paste, and pulp, season with salt and pepper, add a ladle of hot water and simmer for at least 45 minutes with the lid on. Once the ragù is ready, add the soy sauce and a pinch of nutmeg and use it to flavor a nice plate of tagliatelle or a delicious lasagna.

STUFFED RAVIOLI
WITH POTATOES, BEANS
AND PESTO

Preparation: 50 min Cooking: 30 min
Total time: 1 hour and 20 min
For: 4 people
ingredients
350 g potatoes 150 g green beans
2 tablespoons basil pesto 120 g
flour 0 120 g durum wheat
semolina
120 g of water
2 tablespoons of extra virgin olive oil
1 pinch of salt
Peeling tools
Dough rolling machine
Cooking!
Peel and dice the potatoes, then boil
them in lightly salted water for 15
minutes or until soft. Drain them
and

Switch to the potato masher while they are hot, then let them cool. In a pan, heat a little oil and cook the green beans covered for about ten minutes, until they are soft.
Knead the dough
In a bowl, mix the flour, semolina and a pinch of salt, then add the oil and water until you get a smooth and homogeneous dough that we knead for a few minutes. Wrap it in plastic wrap and let it rest at room temperature for an hour. We prepare the filling
Coarsely chop the beans with a knife and combine them with the potatoes along with the pesto, mixing well to combine all the ingredients.

We form the ravioli
With the help of the special machine, roll out
the dough into sheets that are not too thin
and place them on a pastry board sprinkled
with semolina. Fill a sheet with a teaspoon of
filling for each ravioli, keeping them at a
distance sufficient to obtain ravioli of the
desired size. Brush the dough with a little
water and cover with a second sheet of pasta,
letting out as much air as possible from the
ravioli. Cut the ravioli with a pastry cutter
and arrange them on a baking tray sprinkled
with semolina. to cook
Boil the ravioli for about 3 minutes
in lightly salted boiling water, then
sauté them in a pan with a drizzle of
oil and herbs to taste and serve hot.

CAULIFLOWER DUMPLINGS SHALLOW

with shallot and hazelnuts
Preparation: 30 min
Cooking time: 60 min
Total time: 1 hour 30 min
Benefits for: 6
people Ingredients
800 g of cauliflower
360 g of flour 1
240 g of durum wheat semolina
6 shallots
400 ml of soy cream
80 g of hazelnuts
A few sprigs of fresh thyme
Salt and pepper
Steam tools
Hand blender Processor
food ball machine
Dough Bake!
First, wash the cauliflower well,
divide it into florets and steam it.

about 30 minutes, until cooked but not too soft. Transfer to a plate and let cool completely. shallot sauce

For the shallot sauce, cut the shallots into thin slices and cook them in a non-stick pan with a drizzle of oil and a pinch of salt for about twenty minutes, adding a drop of water from time to time if they become too dry. When they are soft, add the soy cream and continue cooking for another 5 minutes. Transfer the mixture to the tall bowl of a blender and blend until smooth and perfectly blended. Season with salt and pepper and set aside. Let's prepare the mixture

Put the cauliflower in the food processor and whisk until smooth. Add the semolina and mix again. Transfer the mixture to a work surface and begin to incorporate the flour a little at a time until it forms a smooth but manageable and no longer sticky dough.

Form the gnocchi

Take one portion of the dough at a time, form a string about 1 cm thick and slice the gnocchi with a small knife.

Roll each gnocchi along the line of lightly floured gnocchi and transfer them as you transfer them to a cutting board or baking sheet dusted with some semolina. Boil and season the gnocchi Once the gnocchi is ready, boil them in a large pot with lightly salted boiling water and drain once they rise to the surface. At this point, sauté your gnocchi in a pan with the shallot sauce, adding a drop of the cooking water from the gnocchi if it is not creamy enough. We serve Serve your gnocchi immediately, garnishing each portion with chopped toasted hazelnuts and a few leaves of fresh thyme.

CHOCOLATE AND ORANGE RISOTTO

Preparation: 10 min Cooking: 20 min
Total time: 30 minutes
For: 4 people

ingredients
360 g of arborio or carnaroli rice
80 g of 85% dark chocolate.
2 tablespoons of unsweetened
cocoa Orange peel
2 shallots
200 ml of white wine
Vegetable broth
1 tablespoon of soy butter (optional)
40 g of chopped walnuts
Cooking!
Finely chop the shallot and brown it in a
high saucepan with a drizzle of oil and a
pinch   of   salt.

When they start to become transparent, add the rice and toast it for a couple of minutes, stirring often to keep it from burning. At this point, blend with the white wine, let it evaporate, then sprinkle with a little boiling broth, adding a ladle at a time as it is absorbed.

We mix the risotto
When the risotto is almost cooked, add the chopped dark chocolate, cocoa, and orange zest and mix well to melt the chocolate completely. Finally, whisk with soy butter, if you wish, and serve your risotto "all'onda", completing each portion with some chopped walnuts.

LASAGNA WITH OLIVES
SCAROLA AND WALNUTS

Preparation: 20 min Cooking: 50 min
Total time: 1 hour 10 min
For 6 people
ingredients
250 g of lasagna without egg
1 kg of escarole
1 onion
1 clove of garlic
750 g of unsweetened soy milk
50 g of flour 0
50 g of olive oil
1 tablespoon of nutritional yeast
60 g of walnuts
80 g of Taggiasca olives
grated vegetable cheese
nutmeg, salt and pepper
Pyrex plate instruments

Cooking!

Start by chopping the onion and brown it in a large non-stick pan or wok with the garlic clove. Cut the endive into strips and wash them well, then drain as much water as possible. Add the salad to the pan and sauté over medium-high heat until softened and some of the water dries. Let's prepare the bechamel

At this point prepare the béchamel: In a saucepan mix the flour with the olive oil and fry for a couple of minutes over low heat, then pour the hot soy milk, continuing to mix with a wooden spoon to incorporate. milk well without lumps. Bring to a boil, turn off the heat,, and season with salt, peit per, nutmeg to taste and nutritional yeast.

boil the lasagna

Meanwhile, bring a pot of water to a boil, lightly salt and pepper and blanch the lasagna for 3 minutes, pouring them a little at a time so that they don't stick. Prepare the lasagna. Spread a spoonful of béchamel on the bottom of the pan, lay a layer of pasta, cover with béchamel, escarole, a few olives, and some coarsely chopped walnuts. Finish by sprinkling with grated vegan cheese and repeat the succession of layers until all the ingredients are used up. Baking

Bake your lasagna in a preheated static oven at 200 ° C for 30 minutes, then remove them from the oven and let them cool for a couple of minutes before serving them sliced.

SEITAN SCALE WITH MUSHROOMS

Preparation: 15 min Cooking: 30 min
Total time: 45 min Servings:
4 ingredients
500 g of seitan 600 g of
mushroom mix ½ leek 1 clove of
garlic 1 tablespoon of chopped
parsley
1 teaspoon of rosemary, chopped
2 tablespoons of cornstarch
2 tablespoons of soy sauce
Vegetable broth Salt e
Cooking pepper.
Let's start by thinly slicing the washed leek
and browning it in a large pan with a drizzle
of oil and the finely chopped garlic clove. In
the meantime, clean the mushrooms very well
and cut them into cubes. Add it to the leeks
and cook over high heat for a couple of
minutes.

Add a ladle of vegetable broth and cook with the lid on for about ten minutes. Brown the seitan In the meantime, cut your seitan into thin slices, cover it with a spoonful of cornstarch and brown it in a pan with a drizzle of oil, it will take 3-4 minutes per side (if necessary you can skip your seitan several times if not everything is ready). Cook the cutlets, blend the mushrooms with the soy sauce, and add the remaining corn starch dissolved in half a glass of water. Cook for a few moments so that the sauce thickens, then add the slices of seitan. Cover with another ladle of vegetable broth and cook for about ten minutes so that the seitan takes on a good flavor.

COOKED VEGETABLES

Preparation: 20 minutes
Cooking time: 25 min
Total time: 45 minutes
For: 4-6 people
ingredients
1 large potato 1 red onion
2 carrots 200 g
cardoncelli mushrooms
300 g of Delicata squash
½ broccoli
150 g of cooked chickpeas
150 g of peas
400 g of tomato pulp
1 clove of garlic
2 bay leaves
2 sprigs of rosemary
1 tablespoon of strong paprika
1 teaspoon of cumin
Vegetable broth
Salt and pepper

Cooking!

First, clean and chop all the vegetables well and divide the broccoli into florets. Cook the vegetables In a large saucepan, fry a little oil with the garlic clove, bay leaf, rosemary, paprika, and cumin, add the chickpeas and all the vegetables except broccoli and peas, and brown for 5 minutes over high heat. Then add the tomato pulp and the vegetable broth, season with salt and pepper, and cook for 10 minutes with the lid on. Complete the goulash Pour the broccoli flowers into the pot and continue cooking for another 10 minutes. Finally, add the peas and cook for another 5 minutes, removing the lid if the goulash is too liquid. Serve your dish hot with slices of toast.

SEITAN ROAST WITH FRIARIELLI AND SUN-DRIED TOMATOES

Preparation: 20 min Cooking: 60 min

Total time: 1 hour and 20 min

For: 4 people

ingredients

160 g of seitan preparation (gluten-free flour)

250 ml of water 300 g of broccoli

10 dried tomatoes in oil

1 teaspoon of rosemary, chopped

1 teaspoon of paprika

¼ , a teaspoon of garlic powder Salt and pepper Vegetable broth 4 tablespoons of soy sauce Cook. Blanch the broccoli for 5 minutes in lightly salted water to soften them, then drain and toss in a pan with a drizzle of oil, salt, and pepper for another 4-5 minutes over medium-high heat to flavor.

We prepare the seitan

In a bowl, mix the gluten flour with the rosemary, paprika, garlic, and a pinch of pepper, then add the water and knead until the dough is smooth and homogeneous. Roll it out on a work surface with the help of a roller until you get a rectangle of about 25 x 20 cm. Distribute the broccoli on the surface of the seitan, forming an even layer and leaving about 1 cm of edge on each side. Also,, arrange the dried tomatoes in two rows and then proceed to roll up your roast starting from the longest side, taking care to seal the edges and ends well. Cook the roast. Wrap the roast in a clean cloth, trying not to squeeze it too much because it will swell a bit during cooking, and close the ends with kitchen twine. Randomly dip into a large pot of boiling, lightly salted broth, drizzle with soy sauce and boil for 50 minutes. Once ready,

VEGAN MEATBALLS WITH PUMPKIN AND POTATOES STUFFED WITH SPINACH

Preparation: 30 minutes
Cooking: 75 minutes
Total time: 1 hour 45 min
For: 8 people
ingredients
750 g pumpkin (weight once cleaned)
250 g potatoes (weight once cleaned)
2 cloves of garlic
1 teaspoon of rosemary, chopped
1 teaspoon of chopped sage
1 tablespoon of nutritional yeast
2 tablespoons of chickpea flour
1 tablespoon of flaxseed flour
250 g of spinach
Cooking!
Start by removing the skin.
and the internal filaments
pumpkin,

Cut it into cubes and cook it in a pan
where you have already heated a
drizzle of oil with rosemary, sage and
garlic.
Season with salt and pepper, complete with a
cover and cook for 20-30 minutes
until it is soft enough
likes to break when crushed
with a fork. cook the potatoes
Meanwhile, peel the potatoes and cut them into
cubes
cubes, then the aromatic herbs in cold water
slightly salty. Once cooked, put
potatoes and pumpkin in a bowl e
mash them with a potato masher
while they are still hot, then leave them
fresh. Let's prepare the spinach
Meanwhile, brown the spinach with a clove
of garlic, a pinch of red pepper, salt and
pepper, just enough time to dry them.
Then transfer them to a colander
and remove as much water as
possible from the vegetation.

Form the meatloaf
Combine the vegetable puree with the
nutritional yeast, the chickpea flour, the
flaxseed flour, and 2 tablespoons of extra
virgin olive oil and mix to incorporate well:
you should obtain a smooth and fairly firm
dough. At this point, roll out the dough on a
baking sheet lined with parchment paper in a
rectangle and place a strip of cooked spinach
in the center. Close the meatloaf with the
help of parchment paper, sprinkle with
breadcrumbs, sprinkle with a drizzle of oil
and fold the meatloaf in parchment paper,
closing the ends with kitchen twine. Cooking
Bake in a preheated static oven at 180 ° C for
30 minutes, then open the parchment paper,
drizzle with another drizzle of oil
y continue cooking for another 15-20
minutes until the surface of the meatloaf is
golden brown. Finally, take it out of the
oven, let it cool for a few moments, and
serve it cut into slices.

FESTIVAL OF VEGAN CAKE

Preparation: 25 min (+ a few hours of resting) Cooking: 50 min Total time: 1 hour 15 min

For: 8 people

ingredients

280 g of flour 2 130 g of raw cane sugar

½ bag of cream of tartar with natural yeast

½ a teaspoon of baking soda

70 g of sunflower oil 280 g of soy milk 2 tablespoons of maple syrup

1 pinch of vanilla powder Zest of an orange 1 pinch of salt for the filling 15 g of cornstarch 150 g of soy milk

30 g of brown sugar 75 g of orange juice 2 tablespoons of rum

1 tablespoon of sunflower oil

1 pinch of turmeric (optional)

for the garnish: 30 g of water

30 g orange juice 2 tablespoons rum 2 tablespoons brown sugar for topping 250 g dark chocolate 75 g soy milk

Tools Grater Cake pan with a diameter of 24 cm Kitchen! First, take care of the base of the cake: pour the flour, brown sugar, baking powder, baking soda, vanilla, salt, and orange zest into a bowl and mix well. Then add the soy milk, oil, and maple syrup and mix all the ingredients until you get a smooth dough. Transfer the dough to a baking tray lined with parchment paper and bake in a static oven at 180 ° C for 40 minutes. Remove the cake from the oven and let it cool completely. Prepare the cream In a saucepan, pour the cornstarch and dilute with a drop of soy milk, then pour in the rest of the milk and add the orange juice, brown sugar, rum, seed oil. and turmeric. Put the saucepan over medium heat and bring the mixture to a boil, continuing to stir with a wooden spoon. Cook for a couple of minutes, turn off the heat and

Transfer the cream to a bowl, covering with cling film. Let the cream cool completely before using it to fill the cake. We fill the cake. For the garnish, mix the water, orange juice, rum, and sugar in a bowl until the sugar has dissolved. With a serrated knife or dental floss cut the cake in half, wet the two halves with the syrup, and fill with the orange cream. Melt the chocolate in a double boiler with the soy milk and pour it on the surface of the cake, reserving a few tablespoons for decoration, if desired. Decorate the cake. Level the chocolate on the surface of the cake well, also covering the sides, then transfer the remaining chocolate into a pastry bag and create the characteristic zigzag lines of the Fiesta.

CAKE WITH CREAM
POTATO
CHOCOLATE DESSERT

Preparation: 30 min Cooking: 40 min
Total time: 1 hour 10 min
For 6 people
ingredients
180 g of flour 2
 20 g of cocoa
50 g of sunflower oil
50 g of maple syrup
30 g of almond milk
1 pinch of yeast 1 pinch of salt
for the filling 120 g of dark chocolate
200 g of cooked sweet potatoes 30 g of
maple syrup
40 g of almond milk
1 teaspoon of cocoa with hazelnut
Cereals Tools Food processing
material Cake pan diameter 18 cm

cooking

Start by peeling the potatoes, cutting them into cubes, sprinkling with sunflower oil and baking them in a preheated static oven at 180 ° C for 20 minutes or until soft. At this point remove them from the oven and let them cool.

We knead the broken dough. For the shortcrust pastry, pour the sifted flour, cocoa, and baking powder into a bowl, add the salt and mix well. Add the seed oil, maple syrup, and almond milk and knead until smooth and smooth. Roll out the shortcrust pastry

Roll out the dough between two sheets of parchment paper with a rolling pin until it forms a disk large enough to cover the bottom and sides of the pan. Lightly grease the mold and place the disc of dough on it, cover it with baking paper, and pour some dried beans or ceramic marbles.

suitable for cooking. We bake in a preheated static oven at 180 ° C for 10 minutes, then remove the beans to cook them in white and continue cooking for another 8 minutes. Then take the base of your cake out of the oven and let it cool completely. We prepare the cream
Blend 200 g of sweet potatoes with a food processor until the mixture is perfectly homogeneous, then add the maple syrup and cocoa and blend again. Melt the dark chocolate
in a water bath, then add the milk almonds and mix well.

most recent,
add the chocolate sauce to the cream
sweet potato
Fill the cake
Immediately transfer the filling onto the ground cocoa mass, leveling the surface well and decorating it with the chopped hazelnuts. Place the tart in the refrigerator for at least an hour to harden the cream, then serve it sliced.

SOFT CORN TACOS WITH SWEET POTATOES, POBLANO AND CORN

serves for 4/6
ingredients

3 tablespoons of extra virgin olive oil
3 cloves of garlic, minced 1½ teaspoon
ground ash 1½ teaspoon ground coriander
1 teaspoon chopped fresh oregano or ¼
teaspoon dried salt 1 teaspoon salt ½
teaspoon pepper 1 sweet potato, mashed,
peeled and chopped, cut into pieces ½
inch 4 poblanos peppers, stemmed and
seeded and cut into ½ inch wide strips 3
ears of corn, kernels deprived 1 large onion,
halved and sliced ½ inch thick
¼ cup fresh cilantro, chopped 12
corn tortillas (6 inches), reheated
Save $

2 ounces of cottage cheese, crumbled (½ cup) 1 quick recipe for shallots and radishes 1 recipe for Mexican cream. Place the oven racks in the upper and lower center position and heat the oven 450 degrees Whisk together oil, garlic, cumin, coriander, oregano, salt, and pepper in a large bowl. Add the potatoes, peppers, corn, and onion to the bowl and toss to coat. Spread the vegetable mixture in an even layer on 2 rimmed baking sheets. Cook the vegetables until tender and golden, for about 30 minutes, stirring the vegetables and flipping and turning the pots halfway through cooking. 3. Return the vegetables to the now-empty large bowl, add the cilantro and stir to combine. Divide the vegetables evenly between the tortillas and decorate with fresh cheese, pickles, and cream. to serve.

PERUVIAN GREEN SAUCE

ingredients

- 2-3 cloves of garlic - 2 green onions -
and half a cup of nonfat sour cream -
and half a bunch of cilantro - chicken
broth (enough to mix) - salt, pepper,
onion powder, chili powder
- low-fat white yogurt (variable in quantity)
- lettuce (optional)
Indications
chop all the ingredients, season, and put
enough chicken broth to mix in a
blender. Taste to see if additional
seasoning is needed. 2. Add yogurt to
lighten the intensity of the sauce's heat
and make it creamier. 3. Refrigerate for
an hour before serving with your favorite
protein or vegetables.

ASPARAGUS IN VIENNA

ingredients

for 4 people:

1 kg of green asparagus
1 stick of butter (200 g)
 4 tablespoons of fine breadcrumbs salt
and pepper Peel the asparagus, wash
them, scrape them gently, and cut them at
the base, removing the woody part; lying
down, tied in bundles, in the asparagus
vase, or in a vase in which they can rest,
immersed for three quarters in water. In
this way they will be able to boil well
without the asparagus heads, which
remain out of the water, running the risk
of darkening and disintegrating.

As soon as they are cooked, gently remove them from the water; Remove the laces and dry them by laying them briefly on a napkin. Then spread them on the bottom of a serving dish and keep them warm while you wait. Now prepare the sauce: melt and heat the butter in a pan. As soon as it is hot, sprinkle the breadcrumbs with salt and pepper and toast it, turning it over and over again with great care so that it does not burn. When they are golden brown, sprinkle the asparagus and serve immediately.

ASPARAGUS WITH LEMON

ingredients
for 4 people
1 kg of Veronese asparagus
1 tablespoon of butter
2 tablespoons of flour
1 egg yolk 100 g of cream
  1 lemon salt and pepper Boil the asparagus;
drain and leave to dry for a few moments on a
napkin. Then transfer them to an oval plate,
arranging them neatly next to each other, all
in the same direction. Then remove the pan
from the heat and pour the cooking water
from the asparagus into the pan. Finally, add
a little salt (if necessary), the finely grated
lemon peel,, and a pinch of pepper. Return
the pot to the heat e Let the liquid thicken
slowly, stirring over low heat until it boils.
Once you have a creamy mixture, add the
egg yolk, cream, and lemon juice little by
little. Pour the sauce over the asparagus and
serve.

ASPARAGUS IN MOUSSELINE SAUCE

ingredients

for 4 people:

800 g of Verona asparagus 4 egg yolks 250 g of butter 1 lemon 60 g of whipped cream 1 tablespoon of mustard salt and pepper Peel the asparagus and boil them in salted water and a lemon wedge; drain them well and put them to dry on a napkin. Meanwhile, put the egg yolks in a saucepan, add two tablespoons of water and place the container in a bain-marie. Do this, beat them with a whisk and beat them. When you have obtained a frothy mixture, gradually incorporate the melted butter (not hot), making it absorb slowly. Finally add the lemon juice, salt and pepper and then the mustard and whipped cream. Spread the sauce on the asparagus in the pan and serve.

POTATO CAKES WITH ASPARAGUS

Ingredients for 4 people:
250 g of mashed potatoes 2 eggs 50 g of flour oil 250 g of wild asparagus 1 glass of milk 1 tablespoon of starch 1 tablespoon of butter 1 clove of garlic 1 sprig of parsley salt and pepper Peel the asparagus, cook and cut into pieces, then sauté them in hot butter with minced garlic. Let them brown slowly, skipping them carefully; then after a few moments add the milk to which starch and a pinch of salt are added; mix and thicken. Then prepare the mashed potatoes; add the finely chopped parsley, beaten eggs, flour, salt and pepper. Fry the mixture in a small greased non-stick pan, dividing it into four portions; then when they are ready Arrange the golden cakes on as many preheated plates and spread on each one a quarter of the hot asparagus cream.

POLISH CAKE OF ASPARAGUS

ingredients
for 4 people:
400 g of asparagus tips 1 liter of milk 250 g
of oat flakes 1 tablespoon of butter 4 eggs
2 tablespoons of grated Parmesan cheese
salt and pepper Pour the milk into a
medium saucepan, put it on the stove,
and bring it to the boil. As soon as it boils,
add the oatmeal and a pinch of salt and
pepper. Lower the heat and let it simmer
for about fifteen minutes. After this time,
turn off the heat, add the butter to the
mixture and let it rest. After a couple of
hours, add the egg yolks to the mixture,
one at a time; then add the egg whites
until stiff, the Parmesan cheese and the
asparagus tips, previously boiled and
well-drained. Pour the mixture into a
greased mold and bake in a preheated
oven at 220 ° for about 25 minutes.

PROVENCAL BARK,

ingredients

for 4 people

200 g of flour 1/2 cup of olive oil
500 g of chard 100 g of black olives 2 onions
2 cloves of garlic 1 sprig of thyme 100 g of
tuma 2 eggs 1 cup of cream 1 knob of butter
salt and pepper Prepare a dough of good
consistency, incorporating the flour, the
olive oil and a little water with a pinch of
salt. Work slowly, then let it rest, wrapped
in a napkin, for about an hour. In the
meantime, clean and bring the pot to a boil;
chopped and browned in a pan with a knob
of butter, chopped olives, onion, garlic and
herbs, salt, and pepper. Let the mixture
cool and add the cheese cut into thin slices
and the eggs beaten with the cream. Roll
out the dough and cut a rectangle; Pour the
chard filling in half and fold to form an
envelope. Seal the edges, rolling up; then
cook the

GRATIN EGGS

ingredients

for 4 people: 600 g of chard 2 cloves of
garlic 2 tablespoons of olive oil 4 large
eggs and 1 yolk 1/2 liter of milk 60 g of
flour 2 tablespoons of white wine vinegar
1 tablespoon of butter 50 g of grated
parmesan salt and pepper Boil the shard;
drain and fry with garlic and oil; then
divide into four buttered cups. Also, dip
the whole eggs in boiling water and
vinegar. As soon as the egg whites are
white and firm, while the yolks are still
soft, drain them with a slotted spoon and
place them in the molds on top of the
vegetables. At this point prepare a thick
béchamel with the milk to which you
have added the butter, flour, and a pinch
of salt. Bring the liquid to a boil, then
quickly add the egg yolk and cheese.

BORAGE FLANGE

ingredients

for 4 people: 400 g of borage 4
tablespoons of olive oil 1 onion 350 g of
fresh ricotta 4 eggs 2 tablespoons of
grated Parmesan cheese 1 knob of butter
1-2 tablespoons of fine breadcrumbs Salt
and pepper Clean the borage by
removing the hard stems , and fry briefly
in a pan with water (just one cup), oil,
chopped onion, salt, and pepper. Let
them cook without a lid for three or four
minutes, then raise the heat and let the
cooking liquid evaporate. Meanwhile,
mix the beaten eggs with the ricotta.
Blend the two ingredients, then mix the
borage with the grated Parmesan, salt,
and pepper. Pour the mixture into a
greased non-stick pan, sprinkle with
breadcrumbs and bake in a preheated
oven at 200 ° for about thirty minutes.

BREAK BROCCOLI

ingredients

for 4 people: 800 g of broccoli florets 1 cup of olive oil 1/2 onion 4 salted anchovies 60 g of black olives 2 tablespoons of grated Parmesan cheese 1 egg yolk 1/2 glass of milk Salt and pepper Peel and clean the broccoli flowers. Boil them in abundant salted water, over high heat and in an uncovered container (to prevent them from turning yellow); drain them and sauté them in a pan with boiling oil, with the chopped onion, turning them carefully several times so as not to crush them excessively. While we turn them, we add the anchovies, desalted, pitted,well-salted, and finely chopped, and the olives, pitted and chopped. Finally, gently level the surface of the preparation. Sprinkle grated Parmesan, dissolved in egg yolk and milk with a pinch of pepper.

PASTRY OF BROCCOLI

Ingredients

for 4 people: 1 pack of frozen puff pastry 400 g of broccoli tapas 150 g of fontina cheese 300 g of stracchino 1 glass of cream or milk 2 eggs salt and pepper While the puff pastry is thawing, peel and boil the broccoli: cook well salted water, over high heat and with an uncovered pot, to prevent them from turning yellow; then drain them. When the broccoli is drained, put it in a bowl and mix it with a well-blended stracchino cream, cream (or milk), fontina cheese, and beaten eggs with salt and pepper. Divide the thawed puff pastry in two and flatten the dough. Place one of the sheets in a greased mold; Pour the broccoli mixture into the cavity and cover with the second leaf, carefully sealing the edges of the two leaves.

ARTICHOKES FROM PIEDMONT

ingredients

for 4 people:

4 Roman-style artichokes 1/2
liter of milk 4 eggs
2 tablespoons of grated Parmesan cheese 1
spring onion 1 tablespoon of butter 100 g of
chicken livers 100 g of beef marrow 100 g of
rooster comb 100 g of veal brains 100 g of
fresh mushrooms 1 glass of dry Marsala
wine broth salt, pepper, and nutmeg Peel
the chopped artichokes and surprise in the
milk with salt and pepper. When they are
tender, put them in the blender with the
eggs, cheese, and cooking liquid and blend
until creamy. Divide the mixture into

four molds and cook in a bain-marie at
180 ° for thirty minutes. In the meantime,
take care of all the meat and mushrooms;
then chop them both carefully and cook
them in a pan with the chopped chives
and butter, salt, pepper, and nutmeg;
halfway through cooking, add the wine
and a little broth. When the puddings are
cooked, we turn over into individual
plates; sprinkle with the spicy meat sauce;
sprinkle with pepper, and serve.

ARTICHOKES WITH OLIVES

ingredients
for 4 people: 4 Roman-style artichokes 40
g of black olives 5 or 6 anchovies in oil 1
cup of olive oil 1 bunch of parsley 1 lemon
Salt and pepper Clean the artichokes by
cutting the ends almost to the heart and
remove the beards by spreading leaves .
Then place them in a pan, arranged
neatly next to each other without
overlapping them, and cook them in a
little salted water and a lemon wedge. As
soon as they are cooked, we drain them
and transfer them to individual saucers,
which we place on slightly larger flat
plates. While it is still hot, sprinkle with
the pitted and chopped olives and the
coarsely chopped anchovies. Season with
an emulsion of oil, lemon juice, salt, and
pepper; sprinkle with chopped parsley
and serve.

CRUSHED ARTICHOKE

ingredients

for 4 people: 6-8 artichokes 1 onion 2
tablespoons of olive oil 6 slices of bacon
120 g of raw ham 2 glasses of milk 75 g
of flour 1 tablespoon of butter
2 tablespoons of Parmesan cheese 1 egg
salt, pepper, and nutmeg Clean the
artichokes; remove the hardest leaves,
tips, and beards; Cut them into thin slices
and sauté them in a pan with a drizzle of
oil, a glass of salted water, and the
chopped onion. Arrange the buttered
slices of bread on the bottom of a
rectangular pan.

Cover with slices of ham; then garnish with the braised artichokes. Once this is done, prepare a thick béchamel with milk, in which a mixture of flour and butter with a pinch of salt has been melted, over moderate heat. As soon as it is thick, add the egg, cheese, pepper and nutmeg. Pour over the artichokes; smooth the surface and place the pan in a hot oven to brown the preparation.

ARTICHOKES IN BARK

ingredients

for 4 people
4 Roman-style artichokes 120 g of
cultivated mushrooms 2 courgettes 1
small white onion 2 cloves of garlic 1/2
cup of olive oil 250 g of frozen puff pastry
150 g of mozzarella 1 lemon 1 tablespoon
of flour breadcrumbs parsley salt and
pepper Put the puff pastry to thaw
naturally in a corner of the work surface
and, in the meantime, peel the
artichokes; Clean and boil them in salted
water, with the flour and a little lemon
juice (to prevent them from darkening).
Separately, cook the zucchini and
mushrooms, cleaned and cut into small
pieces, in a

a drizzle of oil, with chopped garlic, onion and parsley, salt and pepper. As soon as they are cooked, thicken the cooking juices with little breadcrumbs; then add the mozzarella cut into flakes. Then drain the artichokes; Spread the leaves, forming a certain cavity in the center of each one, and pour the mixture of mushrooms and zucchini into the cream. Roll out the dough finely and cut it into four squares. Enclose a stuffed artichoke inside each one; then place the gnocchi in the pan and bake at 190 ° until golden brown.

ANCONA ARTICHOKES FRITTERS

ingredients

for 4 people
100 g of flour 1 egg 1 glass of milk 1
tablespoon of butter 2 or 3 common
artichokes 2 leeks 200 g of fresh pecorino
120 g of raw ham 2 tablespoons of oil salt
and pepper In a medium bowl mix the
egg yolk with the flour and a little
spoons of milk. Once a homogeneous
mass is obtained, dilute with the rest of
the milk; season with salt, and leave to
rest. After a couple of hours, add the
beaten egg white to the mixture. While
the dough rests, peel the artichokes and
surprise them

in a pan, in the oil, with the chopped leeks and one or two tablespoons of salted water.

Grease a pan; Heat over regular heat and brown the fluid batter, two tablespoons at a time. Quickly brown each crepe on both sides; then, taking them with a spatula, quickly transfer them to the oven grill. Stuff immediately with a slice of ham, a spoonful of artichoke mixture, and a triangle of cheese. Fold into a crescent shape and secure with a toothpick. Sprinkle moderately with pepper and bake for a few moments in a hot oven.

CROQUETTES WITH ARTICHOKES

Ingredients for 4 people: 8 common artichokes 3 eggs 2 cloves of garlic oil 1 bunch of parsley flour to taste 1 lemon 400-500 g peanut oil breadcrumbs salt, pepper and nutmeg Clean the artichokes, rub them with the lemon wedge and cut them into small pieces and sauté them in a pan with a drizzle of oil, minced garlic, and parsley, salt and pepper. As soon as they are cooked, pass them through a colander and handle the puree, incorporating the beaten eggs with salt, pepper, and nutmeg and the breadcrumbs necessary to give the preparation a consistency that allows you to take small portions and make lots of meatballs. the size of the nuts. When they are ready, flour them around them, placing them between floured palms; then fry them in abundant boiling oil and serve hot, with lemon wedges and parsley sprigs.

FAGOTTINI WITH ARTICHOKES AND SHRIMPS

ingredients

for 4-6 people
200 g of flour 2 tablespoons of olive oil 2 eggs and 1 yolk 200 g of peeled prawns 1 bunch of parsley 4 common artichokes 2 cloves of garlic 1 bunch of herbs 2 cups of bechamel Milk to taste Salt and pepper In a mixing bowl flour with olive oil, two beaten eggs, a pinch of salt and enough milk to give the dough the consistency of the dough. Beat it with care; then set it aside to rest for a couple of hours. In the meantime, clean the artichokes; Cut them into thin wedges, and brown in a pan with chopped garlic and parsley, a drizzle of oil, salt, and pepper.

Also boil the prawns in salted water, with the bouquet of aromatic herbs, drain and add them to the artichokes, mixing everything with a glass of bechamel. Collect the dough and brown it in spoons in a large greased non-stick pan, brushing it with the back of a spoon, in order to obtain as many round pancakes as possible, as thin as possible. At the end of the preparation of the pancakes, place a spoonful of artichoke and prawn mixture on each one. Roll up, forming cannoli, and place them in a rectangular pan, one next to the other; Paint them with the remaining béchamel, to which you added the egg yolk, and brown in the oven. Serve hot.

ARTICHOKE AND SWITZERLAND FOCACCIA DI BEETS

ingredients

for 4-6 people the following: 1 pack of frozen savory shortcrust pastry 4 artichokes 200 g of chard 400 g of fresh ricotta 2 tablespoons of grated Parmesan cheese 2 eggs 1 bunch of parsley oil milk to taste salt pepper and nutmeg once the mixture has thawed, divide it into two parts. Flatten them both and place the larger of the two in a greased pan about 22cm in diameter. Pour into the cavity of the mass a well-blended mixture of ricotta, milk, beaten eggs, blanched, drained and chopped beets, boiled and chopped artichoke bottoms, grated parmesan, nutmeg, chopped parsley, a tablespoon of oil, salt, and pepper. Cover the filling with the second disc of dough. Seal the edges and place the pan in a preheated oven at 200 °,

EASTER DOOR

ingredients

For 6 people:
4 Roman-style artichokes 800 g of floury potatoes
3 eggs 1 bunch of parsley 2 tablespoons of grated
Parmesan cheese 200 g of cooked minced meat 1
onion 4 tablespoons of olive oil 160 g of stewed
bacon salt and pepper Boil the potatoes; petals
and pass through a colander; Add two beaten eggs
to the puree, a little chopped parsley, Parmesan,
minced meat and bacon, salt and pepper. Spread
the well blended mixture on a rectangle of
aluminum foil and let it wait.

Clean the artichokes; Cut them into slices and sauté them in a pan with oil, chopped onion, and chopped parsley, salt, and pepper. When the artichokes are cooked, add the remaining egg and let it thicken; then let them cool. As soon as they have cooled, place them in the center of the potato mixture. Roll it up and after sealing it inside the film, bake at 200 ° for about half an hour.

SANDIA PIZZA

Preparation time:
10 minutes Servings:

INGREDIENTS 9 oz watermelon slice 1 tablespoon pomegranate sauce 2 oz crumbled feta 1 tablespoon chopped fresh coriander PREPARATION Place the watermelon slice on the plate and sprinkle with crumbled feta. Add the fresh cilantro. After this, generously sprinkle the pizza with pomegranate juice. Cut the pizza into portions. NUTRITION: 143 calories, 6.2 fats, 0.6 fibers, 18.4 carbohydrates, 5.1 proteins

MORNING PIZZA WITH SPROUTS

Preparation time: 15 minutes
Cooking time: 20 minutes
Portions:
INGREDIENTS
½ cup whole wheat flour 2 tablespoons softened butter 1⁄4 teaspoon baking powder 3⁄4 teaspoon salt 5 ounces boiled chicken filet 2 ounces grated cheddar cheese 1 teaspoon tomato sauce 3 ounces bean sprouts
PREPARATION Prepare the pizza dough: mix the wheat flour, butter, yeast and salt. Knead the dough smooth and non-sticky. If necessary, add more wheat flour. Let the dough cool for 10 minutes. Then lay the dough on the baking paper.

Cover with the second baking sheet with parchment paper. Roll out the dough with the help of a rolling pin to obtain the round pizza dough. After this, remove the pan on top of the parchment paper. Transfer the pizza dough to the pan. Spread the cake with tomato sauce. Then cut the chicken filet and place it on the pizza. Add the grated Cheddar cheese. Bake the pizza for 20 minutes at 355 F. Then cover the cooked pizza with the bean sprouts and cut into wedges. NUTRITION: 157 calories, 8.8 fats, 0.3 fibers, 8.4 carbohydrates, 10.5 proteins

CAULIFLOWER FRITTATA

Preparation time: 10 minutes Cooking time: 10 minutes Servings: 2 **INGREDIENTS** 1 cup of chopped cauliflower 1 beaten egg 1 tablespoon of wholemeal flour 30 g of grated Parmesan cheese ½ teaspoon of ground black pepper 1 tablespoon of canola oil **PREPARATION** In the glass of blender, add the grated cauliflower and egg. Add the wheat flour, grated Parmesan cheese and ground black pepper. Mix the mixture with the help of a fork until smooth and without lumps. Pour the canola oil into the pan and bring it. Prepare the pancakes from the cauliflower mixture with the help of your fingertips or with the help of a spoon and transfer them to the hot oil. Grill the pancakes for 4 minutes on each side over medium-low heat. **NUTRITION:** 167 calories, 12.3 fat, 1.5 fiber,

CREAMY OAT FLOUR WITH FIGS

Preparation time: 10 minutes Cook
Time: 20 minutes Servings: 5

INGREDIENTS 2 cups of oatmeal 1 1 ½
cup of milk 1 tablespoon of butter 3 eggs,
chopped 1 tablespoon of honey
PREPARATION Pour the milk into the
saucepan. Add the oatmeal and close the
lid. Cook the oatmeal for 15 minutes over
medium-low heat. Then add the chopped
figs and honey. Add the butter and mix
the oats well. Cook for another 5 minutes.
Close the lid and let the cooked breakfast
rest for 10 minutes before serving.
NUTRITION: 222 calories, 6 fats, 4.4
fibers, 36.5 carbohydrates, 7.1 proteins

PUMPKIN BOAT

Preparation time: 10 minutes Cook
Time: 10 minutes Servings: 4

INGREDIENTS 2 cups of rolled oats 2
cups of water ½ teaspoon of salt 1
tablespoon of butter 1 grated courgette ¼
teaspoon of ground ginger
PREPARATION Pour the water into the
saucepan. Add the oat flakes, butter and
salt. Gently mix and start cooking the
oatmeal for 4 minutes over high heat.
When the mixture reaches a boil, add the
chopped ginger and grated zucchini. Mix
well. Cook the oatmeal for another 5
minutes over medium-low heat.
NUTRITION: 189 calories, 5.7 fats, 4.7
fibers, 29.4 carbohydrates, 6 proteins

SPANAKOPITA BREAKFAST

Preparation time: 15 minutes

Cooking time: 1-hour Servings: 6

INGREDIENTS 2 cups spinach 1 white onion, diced ½ cup fresh parsley 1 tsp minced garlic 3 oz crumbled feta cheese 1 tsp ground paprika 2 eggs, beaten 1/3 cup melted butter 2 oz puff pastry

PREPARATION Separate the phyllo dough into 2 parts. Grease the saucepan well with the butter and put 1 part of the phyllo dough inside. Brush its surface with butter as well.

Put the spinach and fresh parsley in the blender. Blend until the mixture is smooth and transfer it to the mixing bowl. Add the minced garlic, feta cheese, ground paprika, eggs, put the spinach mixture in the saucepan, and flatten well. Coat the spinach mixture with the remaining Phyllo batter and pour the remaining butter over it. Cook the spanakopita for 1 hour at 350 F. Cut into portions.

NUTRITION: 190 calories, 15.4 fats, 1.1 fibers, 8.4 carbohydrates, 5.4 proteins

POBLANO FRITTATA

Preparation time: 10 minutes Cooking time: 15 minutes Servings: 4

INGREDIENTS 5 beaten eggs 1 raw chopped poblano pepper 30 g chopped shallot 1/3 cup cream ½ teaspoon of butter ½ teaspoon of salt ½ teaspoon of chili flakes 1 spoonful of chopped fresh chili with coriander **PREPARATION** Mix the eggs with the cream and beat until a homogeneous mixture is obtained. Add the chopped red pepper, shallot, salt, red pepper flakes, and fresh coriander. Pour the batter into the pan and let it melt. Add the egg mixture and mash it in the pan if necessary. Close the lid and cook the omelet
15 minutes over medium-low heat. When the tortilla is cooked, it will be solid.
NUTRITION: 131 calories, 10.4 fat, 0.2 fibers, 1.3 carbohydrates, 8.2 proteins

PAN OF EGGS AND MUSHROOMS

Preparation time: 7 minutes Cooking time: 25 minutes Yield: 3

INGREDIENTS ½ cup chopped mushrooms ½ chopped yellow onion 4 beaten eggs 1 tablespoon of grated coconut ½ teaspoon of chili 30 grams of grated cheddar cheese 1 teaspoon of canola oil **PREPARATION** Pour the canola oil into the pan and preheat well. Add the mushrooms and onion and cook for 5-8 minutes or until the vegetables are golden brown. Transfer the cooked vegetables to the saucepan. Add the coconut flakes, chili, and cheddar cheese. Then add the eggs and mix well. Cook the casserole for 15 minutes at 180 ° C. **NUTRITION:** 152 calories, 11.1 fats, 0.7 fibers, 3 carbohydrates, 10.4 proteins

GREEN SMOKE FROM BREAKFAST

Preparation time: 7 minutes
Servings: 2

INGREDIENTS
2 cups of spinach 2 cups of kale
curly 1 cup Chinese cabbage 1 ½ cup
almond milk biological one
spoon of almonds minced ½
glass of water
PROCEDURE Put all the
ingredients in the blender and mix
until the mixture is smooth. Pour the
smoothie in serving glasses. Add
ice cubes if you like.
NUTRITION: 107 calories, 3.6 fat, 2.4
fiber, 15.5 carbohydrates, 4.8 proteins

FAST AND SIMPLE STEAK

Preparation time: 15 minutes Cooking time: 10 minutes Servings: 2 INGREDIENTS 1/2 pound steak, quality sliced Salt and freshly ground black pepper INSTRUCTIONS Turn on the fryer, place the basket in it, then set its temperature to 150 ° C and leave to preheat. Meanwhile, prepare the steaks, season the steaks with salt and freshly ground black pepper on both sides. When the fryer has preheated, add the prepared filets to the fryer basket, close with a lid, and cook for 15 minutes. When finished, transfer the steaks to a plate and serve immediately. For meal prep, divide steaks evenly between two heat resistant containers, close with a lid and refrigerate for up to 3 days until ready to serve. When ready to eat, microwave steaks until hot, then serve. NUTRITION: 301 calories, 25.1 total fats, 0 total carbohydrates, 19 proteins.

PANCAKE RICH IN PROTEIN BLENDER

Preparation time: 5 minutes Cooking time: 10 minutes Servings: 1 ingredient 2 organic eggs 1 tablespoon protein powder Salt to taste 1/4 teaspoon cinnamon 2 ounces cream cheese, softened 1 teaspoon unsalted butter INSTRUCTIONS Break the eggs in a blender, add the other ingredients except for the butter and blend for 2 minutes until well blended and blended. Take a pan, put it on medium heat, add the butter and when it has melted pour the prepared batter, distribute it evenly and cook for 4-5 minutes on each side until golden brown. Serve immediately. NUTRITION: 450 calories, 29 g of total fat, 4 g of total carbohydrates, 41 g of protein

BLUEBERRY AND VANILLA LEAVES

Preparation time: 10 minutes Time cooking time: 10 minutes Yield: 12 INGREDIENTS 1½ cup of almond flour 3 organic beaten eggs 2 teaspoons of baking powder

½ cup of stevia 2 teaspoons vanilla extract, unsweetened 3/4 cup fresh raspberries 1 tablespoon olive oil PREPARATION Turn on the oven, then set its temperature to 150 ° C and let it preheat. Take a large bowl, add the flour and eggs, add the yeast, stevia and vanilla until they are well blended, then add the berries until they are well blended. Take a pan, greased with oil, pour over the mixture prepared with a scoop of ice cream, and bake for 10 minutes until cooked. When cooked, transfer the sandwiches to a wire rack, allow them to cool completely, and serve. NUTRITION: 133 calories, 8 g of total fat, 4 g of total carbohydrates, 2 g of protein

AVOCADO EGGS AND
TACOS FOR BREAKFAST

Preparation time: 10 minutes Cooking time: 13 minutes Yield: 2 INGREDIENTS 4 organic eggs 1 tablespoon unsalted butter 2 low-carb tortillas 2 tablespoons of mayonnaise 4 sprigs of coriander ½ sliced avocado Salt and freshly ground black pepper, flavored 1 tablespoon of Tabasco HOW TO USE Take a bowl, break the eggs and beat well until the mixture is homogeneous. Take a pan, put on medium heat, add the butter and when it melts, pour the eggs, distribute them evenly in the pan and cook for 4-5 minutes until cooked.

When cooked, transfer the eggs to a plate and set aside until needed. Add tortillas to pan, cook 2-3 minutes per side until hot, then transfer to plate. Whip the tacos and, for this, spread the mayonnaise on the side of each tortilla, then distribute the cooked eggs and decorate with sliced cilantro and avocado. Season with salt and black pepper, season with Tabasco sauce, and roll up the tortillas. Serve immediately or refrigerate for up to 2 days until ready to eat. **NUTRITION: 289 calories, 27g of total fat, 6g of total carbohydrates, 7g of protein**

PORTOBELLO CAPRESE MUSHROOMS WITH CHEESE

Preparation time: 5 minutes Cook time: 15 minutes Servings: 2

INGREDIENTS 2 large caps of grilled portobello mushrooms 4 tomatoes cut in half Salt and freshly ground black pepper, to taste ¼ cup of fresh basil 4 tablespoons of olive oil ¼ cup of grated mozzarella

INSTRUCTIONS Turn on the oven, then set its temperature to 400 ° F and let it preheat.

Meanwhile, prepare the mushrooms and, to do this, brush them with olive oil and set aside until needed. Put the tomatoes in a bowl, season with salt and black pepper, add the basil, drizzle with oil and mix until smooth. Spread the cheese evenly on the bottom of each mushroom, then cover with the prepared tomato mixture. Take a baking tray, lined with aluminum foil, lay the prepared mushrooms on top, and bake for 15 minutes until completely cooked. Serve immediately. **NUTRITION: 315 calories, 29.2g of total fat, 14.2g of total carbohydrates, 4.7g of protein, 10.4g of sugar, 55 mg of sodium**

CREAMY SOUFFLÉ WITH PARSLEY

Servings: 2 Preparation time: 25 min
INGREDIENTS 2 chopped fresh red chilies Salt to taste 4 eggs 4 tablespoons of cream 2 tablespoons of chopped fresh parsley PREPARATION Preheat the oven to 180 ° and grease 2 soufflé dishes. Combine all ingredients in a bowl and mix well. Pour the mixture into the prepared souffle dishes and transfer it to the oven. Cook for about 6 minutes and unmold to serve immediately. To prepare the food, you can refrigerate this creamy parsley souffle in molds covered with aluminum foil for about 2-3 days. NUTRITION: Calories: 108 Fat:
9 g of carbohydrates:
1.1 g of protein: 6 g of sugar: 0.5 g of sodium:
146 milligrams

PUMPKIN STUFFED WITH BEEF

Preparation time: 45 'Cooking time: 20' INGREDIENTS for four people: 6 fairly large courgettes 4 tablespoons of breadcrumbs 200 g of minced meat 6 thin slices of emmental 1 egg oil 2 tablespoons of milk Clean the courgettes and blanch for 5 minutes in boiling water, then cool and cut in half lengthwise: gently empty the pulp. Chop the zucchini pulp and put it in a bowl, then add the meat, milk, egg, and breadcrumbs, mix and fill the zucchini with the mixture. Place a thin slice on each courgette, sprinkle with breadcrumbs, put everything in a pan, and drizzle with oil. Bake in a preheated oven at 180 degrees for about 20 minutes and serve.

RIGATONI WITH MEATBALLS

Preparation time: 1 hour Cooking time: 10'INGREDIENTS for four people: 400 g of rigatoni breadcrumbs 600 g of tomato pulp 1 egg 200 g of peas 70 g of grated Parmesan cheese 250 g of minced meat garlic 1 onion salt 2 carrots oil butter In a bowl mix the meat and the breadcrumbs , Parmesan and egg: add salt and mix the ingredients. Form small meatballs and brown them in three tablespoons of oil seasoned with a clove of garlic. When they are golden, we reserve them, add another two tablespoons of oil and one of butter to the cooking juices, soften the chopped onion, and add the tomato pulp, season with salt, leave on the stove for 10 minutes, and then add the meatballs. . Cook over low heat for 20 minutes. Boil the diced carrots and peas and, in the meantime, bring the rigatoni to a boil.

ZITI SEA AND MOUNTAIN

Preparation time: 1 hour
cooking: 10'INGREDIENTS for four
people: 400 g of ziti 300 g of tomato pulp
1500 kg of mussels 1 clove of garlic 250 g
of octopus oil 250 g of peeled prawns
half a glass of dry white wine 300 g of
porcini mushrooms salt 1 shallot Clean
the mushrooms and cut them into strips,
chop the shallot and garlic and open the
mussels over medium heat, then peel
them. Clean the octopuses and cut them
into pieces.

In a pan with four tablespoons of oil, brown the shallot and garlic, add the octopus and prawns, brown for 3 minutes, remove and set aside. In the same pan put the tomato pulp, add salt and cook for 10 minutes. In a pan, brown the mushrooms in two tablespoons of oil for 3 minutes. Lightly sprinkle with pepper. Add the octopus, prawns, mushrooms and mussels to the tomatoes and cook for 1 minute. Meanwhile, boil the divided ziti in plenty of boiling salted water and season them.

LASAGNA MAREMMA

Preparation time:
3 hours Cooking time: 30

INGREDIENTS

for four people: egg pasta prepared for lasagna laurel 800 g of bechamel oil 500 g of wild boar meat salt 1/2 liter of Morellino di Scansano wine flour 3 carrots tomato paste 2 onions 50 g of butter 150 g of parmesan celery Marinate the wild boar meat in wine for one night with the vegetables, bay leaf, and a few peppercorns. Drain the marinade and brown the vegetables in four children of oil, add the meat and brown it too, add the salt, two tablespoons of flour, the wine and three tablespoons of tomato paste. Cover and cook for
2 hours. Chop the meat with the cooking juices, grease a baking tray and stuff with layers of lasagna, minced meat, bechamel, and parmesan. Cover with the flakes of butter and bake in a preheated oven at 220 ° for half an hour.

BEAN SOUP
STYLE OF THE HAT
Preparation time: 30′
Cooking time: 20′

INGREDIENTS for four people: 300 g of potatoes 4 chives 350 g of beans in candied chili sauce 1 liter of vegetable broth 3 red peppers oil 3 yellow peppers salt Toast the peppers for a few minutes on the grill, mash them and remove the filaments and seeds: cut into small pieces. Slice the chives and fry them in a saucepan for 3 minutes with four tablespoons of oil, then add the sliced potatoes, yellow peppers, broth and cook over medium heat for 20 minutes. Blend the resulting soup and season with salt. In another saucepan, heat the beans with the red peppers: put the soup in individual bowls and put a spoonful of beans and peppers in each one.

CAKE FOR THE LIPS

Preparation time: 15 '
Cooking time: 45'

INGREDIENTS f

o four people: 1 kg of potatoes 2 tablespoons of breadcrumbs 300 g of anchovy filets 3 onions 23 dl of liquid cream Wash and peel the potatoes and cut them into strips. In a pan, fry the onions cut into strips. Grease a pan, form the first layer of potatoes, cover with anchovy filets and then a layer of onions: continue like this until all the ingredients are used up. Sprinkle the surface with cream, breadcrumbs, and a few flakes of butter. Bake in a preheated oven at 200 ° for 45 minutes.

AGRICULTURAL STYLE

DITALLINE

Preparation time:

1 hour and 30 minutes.

INGREDIENTS

for four people: 150 g of thimbles 20 g of dried mushrooms 50 g of broad beans 2 sprigs of rosemary 50 g of chickpeas olive oil 50 g of lentils 30 g of grated pecorino 50 g of cannellini beans Salt stalk of celery pepper 1 onion Soak the legumes in water in separate containers, soak the mushrooms in warm water and cut the celery and onion into thin slices. Put the chickpeas, rosemary, celery, and onion in a saucepan, cover with water and cook for an hour. Then add the other legumes and continue cooking for another half hour. Season with salt, add the mushrooms, sprinkle moderately with pepper and cook for another 45 minutes. Meanwhile, boil the thimbles in salted water, add them to the legumes,

POLENTA AND MUSHROOMS

Preparation time:
1 hour Cooking time: 30 '

INGREDIENTS

for four people: 500 g of mixed valsugana polenta oil 800 g of butter with mushrooms 20 g of dried mushrooms salt 1 clove of garlic pepper Soak the dried mushrooms in water and clean the mushrooms, which you will cut into slices. In a pan with five tablespoons of oil, brown the garlic, add the dried mushrooms and after 3 minutes the mushrooms, season with salt and pepper, and cook for about 10 minutes. Prepare the polenta, grease a loaf pan, and pour a third of the mixture according to the instructions, spread over half of the mushrooms, make another layer of polenta and then the mushrooms, finally finish with the remaining polenta. Bake in a preheated oven at 180 ° for half an hour and serve.

MARINE POLENTA CAKE

Preparation time: 1 h 30 'Cooking time: 20' INGREDIENTS for four people: 500 g of polenta valsugana dry white wine 500 g of soaked cod, boneless, bay leaf 150 g of sage cream 200 g of shallot oil 4 filets anchovies salt bread crumbs grated parmesan pepper Prepare the polenta according to the instructions and let it cool. Cut the shallot and brown it in four tablespoons of oil with the chopped anchovies, a bay leaf, and a little sage. Add the chopped cod, brown, deglaze with half a glass of wine, let it evaporate, and cover with hot water. Cook for 30 minutes, then add the cream, salt, and pepper and continue cooking for another half hour. Prepare the cake by alternating sheets of polenta and cod in a greased mold.

CREPE DI TREVISO

Preparation time: 45′
Cooking time: 15′

INGREDIENTS for four people: 8 pancakes 100 g of bechamel 400 g of chicory 50 g of butter 150 g of Taleggio oil 150 g of grated Parmesan cheese salt 1 egg pepper 1 shallot **Peel the chicory and cut into strips. Finely chop the shallot and brown it in a pan with three tablespoons of oil, add the radicchio and cook for 3 minutes, then put the mixture in a bowl, add the egg, parmesan, béchamel, and diced taleggio, salt, pepper, and mix well. . Spread the mixture on each pancake, form 8 packs, mix with a little butter and arrange in a greased pan. Bake in a preheated oven at 180 degrees for 15 minutes.**

SOFT PEN

Preparation time:
1 hour and 30 minutes.

INGREDIENTS for four people: 400 g of giant penne 1 clove of garlic 600 g of fresh borlotti beans 4 tablespoons of grated Parmesan cheese 600 g of red tomatoes 1 teaspoon of sugar 1 onion oil 1 carrot salt 1 stalk of celery Peel the beans, put them in cold water and cook for 45 minutes. Chop the onion, carrot, celery, and garlic and brown them in a pan with two tablespoons of oil for 5 minutes. Season with salt, add two tablespoons of bean cooking water, and add the chopped tomatoes. Cook for 10 minutes. Drain the borlotti beans, add them to the sauce, add the sugar and continue cooking for another 20 minutes over low heat. Boil the penne in abundant salted water, drain when al dente, and season with the sauce and Parmesan.

PATIO PENS

Preparation time: 45′
Cooking time: 12′

INGREDIENTS for four people: 400 g of penne 150 g of rocket 2 chicken breasts oil 500 g of tomato pulp salt 2 shallots Finely chop the shallot and brown it in three tablespoons of oil, then add the tomato pulp. Cut the chicken breast into strips and brown it in a pan with two tablespoons of oil, then add it to the pan with the tomato. Boil the penne and a minute before they are cooked add the rocket cut into small pieces: drain the pasta and the rocket, season with the prepared sauce and serve.

ROAST TURKEY

ingredients

750 g of turkey breast
1 glass of dry white wine
100 g of speck
2 cloves of garlic
50 g of butter
salt and pepper
250 g of mascarpone
5 tablespoons of mustard
Preparation
Discover with us all the steps to
make an appetizing baked
turkey breast.
Before starting to prepare the recipe, it is
important to take a little trick to get the
best result: make sure you remove the
mascarpone from the fridge about 30
minutes before preparation.
1 To prepare the turkey in the oven,
preheat the oven to 180 degrees. Take
the turkey breast and sprinkle it with
the
slices   from   speck.

2 Tie the rump with kitchen twine to make it compact, then take a pan and melt the butter; brown the turkey on all sides together with the crushed garlic. 3
Transfer the turkey and butter to a pan, season with salt and pepper. Add the wine and cook for 45 minutes. 4 In the meantime, take a bowl, pour the mascarpone and mix it together with the mustard until you get a smooth and homogeneous cream.
5 Once the turkey is cooked, place it on a cutting board, remove the string and cut it into slices about 1 cm thick. Serve your baked turkey with the freshly made sauce.

Made in the USA
Middletown, DE
30 May 2022

66428033R00159